CH00493036

Diagnosis of the Ort

Diagnosis of the Orthodontic Patient

F. McDonald
Senior Lecturer and Honorary Consultant in Orthodontics,
UMDS Guy's Hospital,
London

and

A. J. Ireland
Consultant Orthodontist,
Royal United Hospital,
Bath

Oxford   New York   Toronto
OXFORD UNIVERSITY PRESS
1998

OXFORD

UNIVERSITY PRESS

Great Clarendon Street, Oxford OX2 6DP

Oxford University Press is a department of the University of Oxford.
It furthers the University's objective of excellence in research, scholarship,
and education by publishing worldwide in
Oxford   New York

Athens Auckland Bangkok Bogotá Buenos Aires Calcutta
Cape Town Chennai Dar es Salaám Delhi Florence Hong Kong Istanbul
Karachi Kuala Lumpur Madrid Melbourne Mexico City Mumbai
Nairobi Paris São Paulo Shanghai Singapore Taipei Tokyo Toronto Warsaw
and associated companies in Berlin Ibadan

Oxford is a trade mark of Oxford University Press
in the UK and in certain other countries

Published in the United States
by Oxford University Press Inc., New York

First published 1998
Reprinted 2000

A catalogue record for this book is available from the British Library

Library of Congress Cataloging in Publication Data
(Data available)

ISBN 0 19 262889 5

Printed in Great Britain
on acid-free paper by
Biddles Ltd., Guildford and King's Lynn

Preface

This book has been written with the specific aim of providing a pocket-sized volume on perhaps the most difficult and yet most enjoyable aspect of orthodontics, diagnosis. It has been inspired by the book *Orthodontic diagnosis* written over 20 years ago by the late Professor W. J. B. Houston, under whose guidance both authors trained in orthodontics. This current book is directed principally at undergraduate dental students, but it is hoped will also be of use to general dental practitioners with an interest in orthodontics and to those embarking on their postgraduate training. The aim is to provide the reader with an understanding of both normal occlusion and malocclusion, and the range of accepted variation. Then, via a logical diagnostic procedure, enable appropriate treatment plans to be reached which fulfil both the patient's needs and expectations.

Included is a chapter on dynamic occlusion. Orthodontists have previously been referred to as 'the masters of the aesthetic malocclusion' and it is necessary that they respect this criticism. All too often the success of orthodontics is decided by the comparison of static models. Legal precedents demonstrate that this is inappropriate in modern-day health care. The book has a chapter on evidence-based practice, as there is currently a greater awareness of the need for treatment to be based on fact, rather than hearsay. Furthermore, orthodontic treatment is not without risk to both short- and long-term oral health and risk/benefit analyses will need to be undertaken in an era of limited resources but increasing expectation and demand. In the later chapters, specimen history sheets are provided along with examples of malocclusions and possible treatment plans. It is not possible to write a book containing treatment plans suitable for each and every circumstance, even though some current weekend postgraduate courses aim to do just that. Various plans of increasing complexity are usually possible for each patient and their presenting malocclusion. For these, the most appropriate for the particular circumstances can be chosen. It is hoped that this book will help the reader both in the determination of possible treatment plans and in choosing the correct course of action for each patient.

London   F.M.
Bath   A.J.I.
December 1997

Acknowledgements

The authors are grateful for the help and assistance of many colleagues in the preparation of this book; in particular Helen Knight, Olga Keith, David Barnett, Bob Mordecai, John Metcalf, Paul Scanlon, Richard Palmer and Chong Weng Lee. We would also like to thank John K. Williams for permission to modify some of the images he created within Harvard Graphics® and Ann Wenzel for allowing us to alter and modify some of her cephalometric illustrations.

Our thanks must also be expressed to all the staff of the Photographic, Printing and Design department of UMDS, London and the Medical Illustration and Photographic Department of the Royal United Hospital, Bath. Both departments have assisted equally in the preparation this textbook.

And, finally, we are grateful to the support of our families for more than one aspect of the preparation of this book.

Contents

CONTENTS

1

Development of the normal dentition

1.1 BIRTH

At birth the deciduous teeth are usually unerupted and the alveoli comprise a thickened mucosal covering known as the gum pads (Fig. 1.1). These are subdivided into raised areas corresponding to the position of the unerupted deciduous teeth, by shallow transverse grooves on the mucosal surface. To the lingual of these raised areas, running around the arch in both the upper and lower jaws, is another shallow groove known as the dental groove. It is from here that epithelial ingrowth originates to form the enamel organ. In addition, in the upper jaw a further shallow groove, known as the gingival groove, passes around the arch palatal to the dental groove. This denotes the boundary between the epithelium of the alveolus and the palate.

The upper gum pad is horseshoe-shaped and overlaps the more U-shaped lower gum pad anteriorly and buccally. The two are rarely brought together, and at rest the tongue will usually lie between them.

A detailed examination of the neonate is usually only required in the case of developmental defects such as clefts of the lip and palate or when natal or neonatal teeth are present.

1.2 DEVELOPMENT OF THE DECIDUOUS DENTITION

Typically, deciduous tooth eruption begins with the lower central incisors at approximately six months of age. The commonly quoted eruption times may vary by plus or minus six months. Thus a lower central incisor may be present at birth and is then referred to as a natal tooth. If it should erupt within the first 30 days after

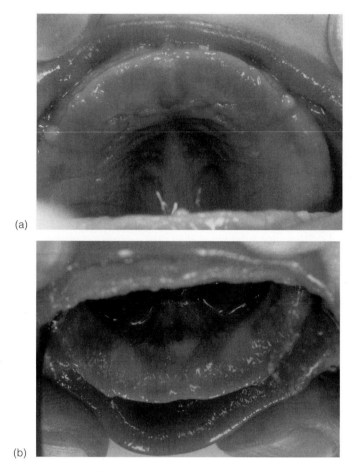

(a)

(b)

Fig. 1.1   Upper and lower gum pads showing elevations corresponding to the unerupted deciduous teeth, as well as the dental and gingival grooves in (a) the maxilla, (b) the mandible.

birth it is referred to as neonatal tooth.[1] These teeth are usually of the normal series but have erupted prematurely.[2,3] As a consequence, formation of both the root and some of the enamel may be incomplete. The teeth can therefore be very mobile, as well as slightly hypoplastic in appearance. If a natal or neonatal tooth is causing problems, most likely with breast feeding, it can be extracted. The decision to leave or extract such a deciduous incisor

Table 1.1 Calcification, eruption, root completion times, and mesiodistal widths of the deciduous dentition

	Calcification complete (months)	Eruption (months) ± 6 months	Root complete (months)	Mesiodistal widths (mm)	
				Maxillary	Mandibular
Central incisor	2–3	6		6.5	4.0
Lateral incisor	2–3	9	12–18	5.0	4.5
Canine	9	18	after eruption	6.5	5.5
First molar	6	12		7.0	8.0
Second molar	12	24		8.5	9.5

needs to be weighed against the need to establish a good, early feeding pattern.

Eruption times are as listed in Table 1.1. It should be noted that the mandibular teeth erupt 1–2 months in advance of their maxillary counterparts.

1.2.1 Normal occlusion

By the age of 30 months all the deciduous teeth should have erupted. A number of characteristic features are usually present, namely:

1. The incisor relationship is such that there is usually a positive overjet and overbite. (See p. 55)
2. The incisors are more retroclined than their permanent successors.
3. Space is usually present mesial to the upper deciduous canines and distal to the lower deciduous canines and is known as primate spacing.
4. Each maxillary tooth occludes with the corresponding mandibular tooth and the one distal to it, with the exception of the upper second deciduous molar.
5. When the second deciduous molars are in occlusion, their distal surfaces lie in the same vertical plane.

1.2.2 Age changes from 3 to 6 years in the normal deciduous dentition

1. Spacing may begin to appear or increase in the labial segments as a result of growth.
2. Occlusal attrition may become evident.
3. The relative incisor position can progress toward a class III incisor relationship (see p. 55), and may even reach an edge to edge occlusion as a result of mandibular growth.
4. The distal surfaces of the second deciduous molars may no longer remain in the same vertical plane.
5. The first permanent molars begin to erupt, usually into a half unit class II molar relationship, guided by the distal surfaces of the second deciduous molars.

Although the above are the classically described age changes, they may not necessarily take place.[4] A factor which is likely to be present in many children at this age and one which will certainly play a major role in the position of the incisor teeth is a digit sucking habit.

1.3 PROGRESSION TO THE MIXED DENTITION

The period of the mixed dentition begins with the eruption of the first permanent molars at approximately six years of age and will end when the last deciduous molar is exfoliated and the permanent dentition becomes established. As in the case of the deciduous dentition the mandibular teeth usually erupt ahead of the corresponding maxillary teeth. Eruption times are given in Table 1.2.

1.3.1 Age changes from 6 to 9 years in the mixed dentition

In the lower arch a typical combined mesiodistal width of the deciduous incisors measures 17 mm, whilst that of their permanent successors is 23 mm. In the upper arch the two measurements are 23 mm and 30 mm respectively. The additional space required in each arch for the permanent incisors comes from three sources:

(1) spacing already present in the deciduous labial segments;

(2) an increase in the intercanine width due to growth as the permanent incisors begin to erupt; and

(3) as the permanent incisors are more proclined they erupt into a larger arc of a circle than the deciduous incisors.

In the lower arch the permanent incisors may erupt lingual to their deciduous precursors and are likely to be crowded. If this occurs the deciduous incisor should be extracted before the permanent tooth attains a reasonable occlusal level. The permanent tooth will then move anteriorly into the arch under the influence of the tongue. Occasionally a lower deciduous canine will be resorbed by an erupting and crowded permanent lower lateral incisor. The resulting shift of the lower centreline to the affected side, which is a reflection of crowding in the permanent dentition, can be prevented by extracting the remaining lower deciduous canine tooth at this time (a balancing extraction).

In the upper arch it is normal for the upper permanent incisors to erupt distally angulated and hence spaced. This spacing has been termed the 'ugly duckling stage' but as it is a normal stage of development is more appropriately termed 'physiological spacing'. It is related to the developmental position of the unerupted upper permanent canines and is the commonest cause of a median diastema, albeit transiently. As the permanent canines erupt this spacing will close spontaneously (Figs 1.2 and 1.3). Other possible causes of a median diastema at this and later stages include:

(1) midline supernumerary (mesiodens);

(2) developmentally absent upper lateral incisors;

(3) small or peg-shaped upper lateral incisors;

(4) small teeth and generalized spacing;

(5) fleshy upper labial frenum;

(6) proclined upper incisors, for example, as a result of a digit sucking habit (see Chapter 2), incompetent lips, or racial factors as in bimaxillary proclination (see Chapter 4);

(7) trauma;

(8) midline cyst (e.g. nasopalatine duct cyst).

If crowding is present in the upper labial segment during incisor eruption, it will result in the upper permanent lateral incisors

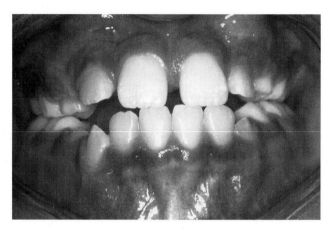

Fig. 1.2 Clinical photograph of a patient aged eight years showing the 'ugly duckling' phase.

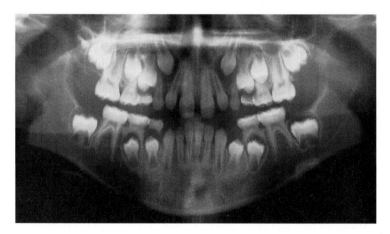

Fig. 1.3 Physiological spacing in the upper labial segment prior to the eruption of the upper permanent canines in a different case to Fig. 1.2 but with enlarged canine follicles. Note the close proximity of the unerupted permanent canines to the roots of the upper lateral incisors.

erupting into a more palatal position than normal. This is due not only to their palatal developmental position but also because they erupt after the upper central incisors and before the upper deciduous canines are shed.

During development of both the deciduous and permanent dentitions, facial growth occurs in all three planes of space. In order that the teeth should remain in occlusal contact during, in particular, vertical facial growth, they continue to erupt once in the mouth. This stage of developmental change often goes unnoticed. However, occasionally the dynamic process of resorption and subsequent repair of the deciduous teeth, which is part of the normal physiological process of shedding, favours repair rather than resorption.[8] The tooth then becomes partially fused to the underlying bone and is said to be ankylosed. It no longer erupts as do the adjacent teeth and so appears to submerge relative to its neighbours. In extreme cases the tooth may become totally submerged, only being visible on radiographic examination.

1.4 THE PERMANENT DENTITION

Subsequent to the eruption of the first permanent molars and incisors, the permanent dentition becomes established with the eruption of the permanent canine and premolar teeth. The final teeth to erupt are the second and third permanent molars.

1.4.1 Age changes from 10 to 12 years in the buccal segments

As in the labial segments there is a difference in the combined mesiodistal widths of the permanent canine and premolars in each quadrant of the mouth compared with their deciduous precursors. The combined mesiodistal widths are given in Tables 1.2 and 1.3.

In both arches the combined mesiodistal width of the three permanent teeth is less than that of the corresponding deciduous teeth and this difference is known as the leeway space. In the deciduous dentition, there is primate spacing distal to the lower deciduous canine and mesial to the upper deciduous canine. No such spacing exists in the permanent dentition. The leeway space is eventually lost as mesial drift of the first permanent molars occurs following the eruption of the permanent canines and premolars. The larger leeway space in the lower arch enables the lower first permanent molar to drift further mesially than the upper first permanent molar. The molar relationship will therefore change from a cusp to

Table 1.2   Calcification, eruption, root completion times, and mesiodistal widths of permanent dentition[2-7]

	Calcification commences (months)	Eruption (years) ± 6 months	Root complete (years)	Mesiodistal widths (mm)
Mandibular				
Central incisor	3–4	6.5		5.5
Lateral incisor	3–4	7.5		6.0
Canine	4–5	10.0		7.0
First premolar	21–24	10.5	2–3 post eruption	7.0
Second premolar	27–30	11.0		7.0
First molar	Birth	6.0		11.0
Second molar	28–36	12.0		10.5
Third molar	8–10 years	18.0		10.5
Maxillary				
Central incisor	3–4	7.5		8.5
Lateral incisor	12	8.5		6.5
Canine	4–5	11.5		8.0
First premolar	18–21	10.0	2–3 post eruption	7.0
Second premolar	24–30	11.0		6.5
First molar	Birth	6.0		10.0
Second molar	30–36	12.0		9.5
Third molar	7–9 years	18.0		8.5

Table 1.3   The combined mesiodistal widths of the deciduous canines and molars and their permanent successors

	Combined mesiodistal widths (mm)	
	Deciduous – C, D, E	Permanent – 3, 4, 5
Mandibular	23	21
Maxillary	22	21.5

cusp relationship in the mixed dentition, seen when their eruption was guided by the coincident distal surfaces of the second deciduous molars, to a class I relationship (see p. 54) in the permanent dentition.

At approximately 12 years of age the second permanent molars begin to erupt. Their eruption into the correct class I relationship is guided by the distal surfaces of the first permanent molars.

1.4.2 Late changes in the permanent dentition

The last teeth to erupt are the third permanent molars. Their eruption time is variable and it is not unusual for there to be insufficient space for them to erupt into an acceptable position within the arch.

A common change in the permanent dentition in the late teens to early twenties is late lower incisor crowding. A number of mechanisms have been proposed to account for this feature, including those listed below.

1. Continued mandibular growth. The combined effect of a mesial translation of the lower buccal segment teeth with growth, and retroclination of the lower incisors under the influence of the lower lip, will cause dental arch shortening, which will manifest itself as lower incisor crowding.

2. Mesial drift. As with late lower incisor crowding itself there are a number of possible theories to account for mesial drift. These include
    (a) the mesial component of masticatory force due to the mesial inclinations of the teeth;
    (b) transeptal fibre contraction – an unlikely cause;
    (c) the mesial eruptive path of teeth.

3. Eruption of the third permanent molars. The eruption of these teeth is another possible cause of mesial drift. However, it is thought unlikely to be a cause of late lower incisor crowding since this can frequently occur in the absence of these teeth.

1.5 IDEAL AND NORMAL OCCLUSION

The ideal occlusion in the permanent dentition has a number of general characteristic features. Skeletal bases should be

(1) of the correct size relative to each other and the teeth; and
(2) in the correct relationship in all three planes of space at rest.

The following occlusal relationships should be observed.

1. All teeth are present and are in correct contact with their immediate neighbours in the same arch with no spacing and/or rotations.

2. There is no tooth size disproportion between the maxillary and mandibular teeth (i.e. the sizes of the upper arch teeth are correct relative to those of the lower arch).

3. The teeth are at the correct inclinations and angulations on their respective skeletal bases (i.e. buccal segment teeth should be slightly mesially angulated and lingually inclined and the labial segment teeth slightly mesially angulated and proclined).

4. Each upper tooth occludes with the corresponding lower arch tooth and the one distal to it, with the exception of the upper third permanent molar.

5. The upper teeth lie labial/buccal to the lower teeth. The lower labial segment teeth therefore occlude with the palatal surfaces of the upper labial segment teeth and the buccal cusps of the lower buccal segment teeth occlude in the fossae of the upper buccal segment teeth.

6. The occlusal plane is slightly curved and can be considered to form part of a sphere with the mandibular teeth occluding on the outside and the maxillary teeth occluding on the inside of this sphere. The curvature in the sagittal plane is known as the curve of Spee, whilst in the coronal plane it is known as the curve of Monson.

7. Both the maxillary and mandibular arches are symmetrical and coordinated with each other.

8. The incisor, canine, and molar relationships are class I (see Chapter 2 for definitions).

In function, the following observations will be made:

(1) on protrusion there is incisal guidance where the incisors remain in contact but the buccal segment teeth do not;

(2) in lateral excursions there is either canine guidance or group function in the buccal segments and there are no balancing or non-working side interferences (see Chapter 6).

Although such occlusion might represent the ideal, it is seldom encountered. More usually there are minor and insignificant variations in some or all of the above features which do not compromise the patient in terms of health, function, or aesthetics. The dentition is a dynamic system and minor changes frequently occur as a consequence of use and ageing. It is therefore better to consider the concept of a 'normal occlusion' in clinical practice, although the precise limits of 'normal' are difficult to define. What might be considered normal to one clinician, and equally important to the patient, might not be considered normal by another. Large variations from normal about which there is no disagreement can confidently be defined as a malocclusion. Normal occlusion is a realistic treatment aim in the correction of any malocclusion and Andrews[9] has defined six 'keys' (derived from an examination of 120 'normal' untreated cases) listed below, which need to be achieved if this aim is to be fulfilled.

1. Correct molar relationship – distal surface of the upper first permanent molar distobuccal cusp occludes with the mesiobuccal cusp of the lower second permanent molar.
2. Correct crown angulation (mesodistal tip of the crown).
3. Correct crown inclination (labiolingual or buccolingual).
4. No rotations.
5. Tight approximal contacts.
6. Flat occlusal plane – this is considered a desirable overcorrection since the curve of Spee is expected to increase with continued mandibular growth.

Summary of development of the normal dentition

The stages of importance in the development of the normal dentition are
(1) birth;
(2) development of the deciduous dentition between 6 and 24 months ± 6 months;
(3) age changes from three to six years of age in the deciduous dentition in preparation for the eruption of the permanent teeth;
(4) the mixed dentition, beginning with the eruption of the first permanent molars;
(5) age changes from six to nine years as the permanent incisors erupt;
(6) age changes from 10 to 12 years principally in the buccal segments as the premolars and also the permanent canines erupt;
(7) the permanent dentition;
(8) late changes in the permanent dentition.

continue on next page

Summary of development of the normal dentition
(continued)

In an ideal occlusion all 32 permanent teeth will be perfectly related to the adjacent and opposing teeth. The concept of a normal occlusion, in which very minor and acceptable irregularities are present, is a more realistic and attainable long-term occlusion following orthodontic treatment.

Objectives

1. Recall all eruption dates
2. List features of an ideal occlusion
3. Outline stages of development of normal occlusion

REFERENCES

1. Massler, M. and Savara, B. S. (1950). Natal and neonatal teeth. Review of twenty four cases reported in the literature. *Journal of Paediatrics*, **36**, 349–59.
2. Southam, J. C. (1968). The structure of natal and neonatal teeth. *The Dental Practitioner*, **18**, 423–7.
3. Berman, D. S. and Silverstone, L. M. (1975). Natal and neonatal teeth. *British Dental Journal*, **139**, 361–4.
4. Foster, T. D., Grundy, M. C., and Lavelle, C. L. B. (1972). Changes in the occlusion in the primary dentition between $2\frac{1}{2}$ and $5\frac{1}{2}$ years of age. *Transactions of the European Orthodontic Society*, 75–84.
5. Logan, H. G. and Kronfield, R. (1933). Development of the human jaws and surrounding structures from birth to the age of fifteen years. *Journal of the American Dental Association*, **20**, 379–427.
6. Schour, I. and Massler, M. (1940). Studies in tooth development: the growth pattern of human teeth. *Journal of the American Dental Association*, **27**, 1918–31.
7. Gorlin, R. J., Pindborg, J. J., and Cohen, M. M. (1976). *Syndromes of the head and neck*, (2nd edn). McGraw-Hill, New York.
8. Scott, J. H. and Symons, N. B. B. (1982). In *Introduction to dental anatomy*, (9th edn), The establishment of the decidous and permanent dentitions, pp. 130–3. Churchill Livingstone, London.
9. Andrews, L. F. (1972). The six keys to normal occlusion. *American Journal of Orthodontics*, **62**, 296–309.

2

Malocclusion: aetiology and classification

2.1 AETIOLOGY OF MALOCCLUSION

The factors involved in the aetiology of malocclusion are numerous but traditionally have been divided into general and local factors. General factors are often quoted as being skeletal factors, soft tissue factors, and habits, whilst dento-alveolar factors are often referred to as local. This division into general and local factors can give the wrong impression as to how each of these aetiological agents act in the production of a malocclusion. For example, the effect on the occlusion of incompetent lips might be limited to proclination of the upper incisors, whilst having no effect on the buccal segment teeth or lower incisors. On the other hand, the dento-alveolar factor of crowding, due to one or more large teeth, is often described as a local factor, yet its effects might be seen throughout the occlusion. For this reason the aetiological factors in the development of malocclusion are best considered as

- skeletal factors
- soft tissue factors
- dento-alveolar factors
- habits.

In order to be able to classify and subsequently plan the treatment of a malocclusion it is necessary to understand the constituent parts involved in its aetiology and how they interrelate to produce the presenting malocclusion. It is not always possible to identify one aetiological factor which, if corrected, would enable treatment of the malocclusion. However, identifying the major factor may help identify the type(s) of treatment required for correction of the malocclusion. Classically for example, large skeletal discrepancies require functional appliances for correction in growing patients and surgical treatment in non-growing, adult patients. Dento-alveolar discrepancies on the other hand usually require more localized treatments.

The aetiology of most malocclusions is multifactorial. Therefore, a systematic approach to examination, diagnosis, and subsequent classification of the malocclusion will help the clinician to establish a mental picture not only of the aetiology but how the malocclusion might be treated.

The role of each factor in the aetiology of malocclusion will now be discussed.

2.1.1 Skeletal factors

Skeletal structures can vary in all three planes of space – antero-posterior, vertical, and transverse. Of all the possible aetiological factors these are almost certainly the easiest to identify and yet are amongst the most difficult to correct.

In initially understanding the effect of any aetiological agent on the occlusion it is often useful to consider its extremes. The role of other aetiological factors can then be overlaid on the effect created by the principal agent. For example, the effect of an adverse antero-posterior skeletal relationship on the occlusion may be modified (Fig. 2.1) by the surrounding soft tissues, leading to changes in the inclination of the teeth. This is known as dento-alveolar 'compensation' (see Glossary) and is a static phenomenon. Orthodontic treatment often involves further modification of tooth position to overcome the effect of skeletal pattern.

Anteroposterior skeletal relationship

Ideally, and in a normal class I (see p. 58) skeletal relationship, the maxillary base should be just ahead of the mandible (Fig. 2.2). In prognathic, or class III cases, the mandible is more anteriorly placed than the maxilla, either because it is larger than the maxilla, or because its articulation with the base of the skull is more anteriorly placed than normal (Fig. 2.3). In the retrognathic or class II skeletal case the opposite is true (Fig. 2.4).

If no dento-alveolar compensation is seen in cases where the skeletal pattern is anything other than class I, then the anteroposterior

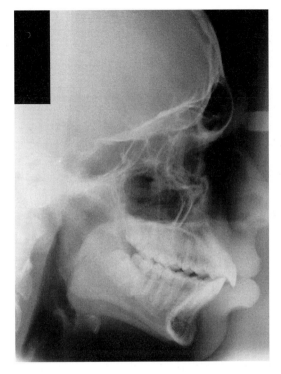

Fig. 2.1 The lateral skull radiograph illustrates how dento-alveolar compensation has occurred in the presence of a class II skeletal pattern. The lower incisors are proclined, reducing what would otherwise be a large overjet due to the adverse skeletal pattern.

relationship of the upper and lower incisors is a true reflection of the underlying skeletal discrepancy (Fig. 2.5). However, it is not uncommon for the soft tissues to modify the inclination of the incisors such that the relationship of the incisors is less than expected by the assessment of skeletal pattern. This can be considered the biological mechanism of creating a class I incisor relationship in the absence of a normal skeletal relationship. As a consequence, many clinicians mentally reposition the upper and lower incisors to their correct inclination over their respective skeletal bases in order to try to visualize the extent of any skeletal discrepancy. This can be performed more accurately by using a tracing of a lateral skull radiograph and is referred to as a Ballard's conversion (see Chapter 8).

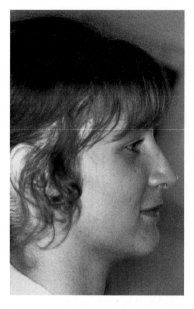

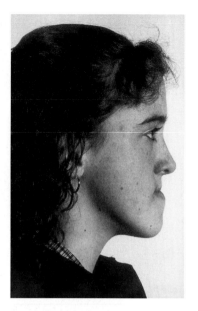

Fig. 2.2 Profile view of patient with a class I skeletal pattern.

Fig. 2.3 Profile view of patient with a class III skeletal pattern.

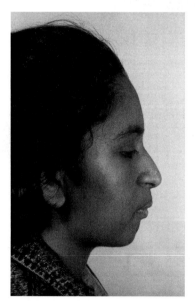

Fig. 2.4 Profile view of patient with a class II skeletal pattern.

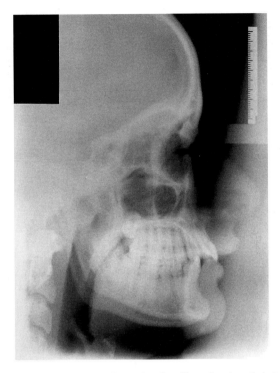

Fig. 2.5 Lateral skull radiograph illustrating the effect of a class II skeletal pattern in producing an increased overjet in the absence of dento-alveolar compensation.

A class II skeletal pattern can be used to illustrate the effect of anteroposterior skeletal pattern on the labial segment teeth and how this can be modified by other factors such as the surrounding soft tissues. If there is a marked class II skeletal relationship and the incisors are unaffected by the soft tissues then the horizontal distance between the upper and lower incisors, or overjet (see Chapter 5), will be a reflection of the underlying skeletal relationship as discussed previously. If, as a result of the retrognathic mandible, the patient's lips at rest do not cover the upper incisors, then the upper incisors may procline. The lower incisors, however, may be retroclined by the lower lip. The discrepancy between the upper and lower incisors is therefore more marked than is suggested by the underlying skeletal malrelationship. The incisor relationship created is known as class II division 1 (see p. 55). It is possible that in such a case the incisor position could be altered by orthodontic treatment to produce a normal incisor relationship, even though the skeletal pattern is not normal (dento-alveolar compensation). If the class II anteroposterior skeletal relationship is less marked than that described, the soft tissues may alter the position of the incisor teeth in a completely different manner. In such a case the lower lip may easily cover the upper incisors at rest and cause them to retrocline (Fig. 2.6). In this case dento-alveolar compensation has produced a different incisor relationship, namely class II division 2.

Similarly, in the case of a prognathic mandible, the overjet may be reduced or reversed and the incisor positions modified by the soft tissues (Fig. 2.7).

The interrelationship between the different aetiological agents involved in the development of a malocclusion can be complex. In any case it is essential to try to understand the action of the principal agent and how its effect can be modified by any others.

Vertical skeletal relationship

In order to understand the effect of variations in vertical skeletal relationship on the development of malocclusion it is once again worth considering what is normal and then considering extremes.

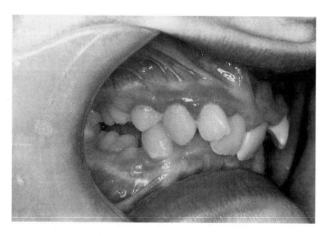

Fig. 2.6   A high lower lip line in this case has caused retroclination of the upper central incisors to create a class II division 2 incisor relationship.

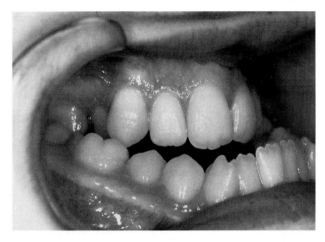

Fig. 2.7 A photograph demonstrating dento-alveolar compensation of the upper and lower labial segment teeth in the presence of a class III skeletal pattern. The lower incisors are retroclined and the uppers are proclined.

A normal vertical skeletal relationship is seen when the height of the anterior lower face, that is, the distance between the base of the chin to the base of the nose, equals the upper anterior facial height, as measured from the base of the nose to the area between the eyebrows (see Chapter 4). In addition, the angle between the lower border of the mandible (mandibular plane) and a line passing between the lower border of the orbit and the upper border of the external auditory meatus (Frankfort plane), known as the Frankfort–mandibular planes angle (FMPA), should be approximately 27° ± 5°. This angle helps in the assessment of the ratio between the anterior lower face height and the posterior lower face height and will be discussed in more detail in Chapter 8.

If there is a mismatch in growth between anterior and posterior facial heights then two extremes of variation of vertical dimension can arise. If the anterior part of the mandible grows downwards, away from the maxilla, and in some cases the anterior part of the maxilla also grows upwards, away from the mandible, the anterior face height might be increased and the patient is said to have a posterior growth rotation (Fig. 2.8). If the opposite occurs it is known as an anterior growth rotation and the anterior lower face height decreases.[1]

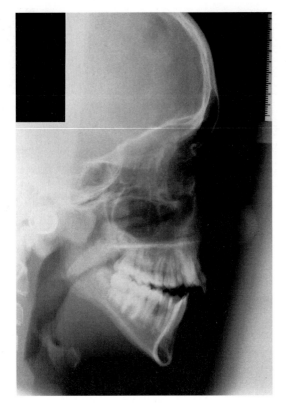

Fig. 2.8 Lateral skull radiograph of a patient exhibiting a posterior growth rotation. Note the pronounced notch on the lower border of the mandible close to the angle, and high maxillary mandibular planes angle (see Chapter 8).

In many ways, consideration of this dimension has typified the change in understanding of present day orthodontics by identifying different facial types and how they might arise.

In patients with a posterior growth rotation the increased anterior lower facial height may produce what is known as a long face. This increase in the anterior vertical skeletal dimension can have a profound effect on the occlusion. In extreme cases the vertical height will exceed the eruptive potential of the labial segment teeth. This may either lead to a reduced vertical overlap of the incisor teeth (overbite) or may indeed mean there is no overlap of the incisors. In the latter instance, it is known as an anterior open bite and when extreme may

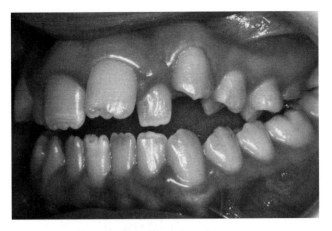

Fig. 2.9   An anterior open bite extending into the buccal segments such that only the second permanent molars are in occlusion.

extend into the buccal segments, such that only the second permanent molars are in occlusion (Fig. 2.9). The fact that the teeth have
reached their maximum eruptive potential will have implications for
treatment. It will not be possible to extrude the incisor teeth to
produce a positive overbite and expect the supporting alveolar bone
to follow. Any attempt at extrusion might compromise the long-term
bony support of the teeth. Treatment should therefore be aimed at
either accepting the open bite or correcting the principal aetiological
agent, namely the vertical skeletal discrepancy.

The converse of this is seen in patients with an anterior growth
rotation, where a square type face with a decreased anterior lower
face height is present. As a consequence of the reduced distance
between the maxilla and the mandible, the labial segments, which
are well within their eruptive potential, may erupt past one
another, unless they are prevented from doing so by the opposing
teeth. As a result there may be an increased overbite. This increased overbite may be complete to the opposing teeth, or in some
cases to the soft tissues of the opposing arch. In this situation the
overbite may not only be deep but also traumatic either to:

- the labial gingivae in the mandible (Fig. 2.10), or
- the palatal gingivae in the maxilla, or
- both of the above.

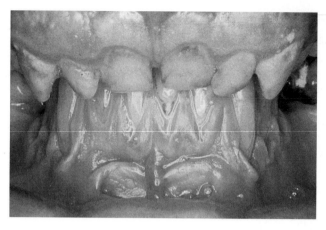

Fig. 2.10 Stripping of the lower labial segment gingivae as a result of a deep traumatic overbite.

From a periodontal viewpoint the degree of trauma can be sub-divided further into four subgroups, types I–IV, as described below.[2]

1. Type I – the mandibular incisors impinge into the palate.
2. Type II – the mandibular incisors impinge into the gingival sulcus of the maxillary incisors.
3. Type III – both maxillary and mandibular incisors are inclined lingually and impinge into the tissues of the opposing arches.
4. Type IV – the mandibular teeth move or extrude into the abraded lingual surfaces of the maxillary teeth.

The effect of vertical skeletal relationship on the occlusion can also be modified by other factors such as the soft tissues. For example, when there is an increased anterior lower face height and increased FMPA, the lower incisors can be found to be retroclined under the influence of what is often a strong and active lower lip. This will be discussed further in Chapters 4 and 8.

One specific type of facial appearance is described as adenoid faces which, as a term, is an inference to the aetiology. The skeletal pattern in this case is typified by a long face with bilateral narrowing of the maxilla. This will be discussed further under the heading 'Soft tissues'.

Transverse skeletal relationship

Typically the maxilla is slightly broader than the mandible, resulting in the correct positioning of the buccal segment teeth as described in Chapter 1. That is, the upper molars and premolars occlude half a tooth width buccal to the corresponding lower arch teeth.

Transverse skeletal discrepancies are either unilateral or bilateral and are often reflected in the position of the buccal segment teeth. They may also be associated with atypical mandibular movements such as a mandibular displacement on closing into centric occlusion (see Chapter 6). The transverse discrepancy may either be due to a mismatch in size between the mandible and the maxilla, or due to an abnormal articulation of the mandible with the cranial base. If the articulation is more anteriorly positioned than normal and yet the size of each jaw is correct, a wide part of the mandible will oppose a narrow part of the maxilla. This may be reflected as an abnormal transverse relationship of the upper and lower buccal segment teeth.

Intra-orally, transverse discrepancies may be seen as either a crossbite (if the maxilla is narrow) or a scissors bite (if the maxilla is wide with respect to the mandible). In the former case the cusps of the upper buccal segment teeth will occlude with the opposing lower arch teeth in an upper buccal cusp, to lower arch occlusal fossae manner in centric occlusion (Fig. 2.11). In the latter case, the upper buccal segment teeth occlude further buccally than normal, sometimes occluding totally outside the opposing mandibular teeth (Fig. 2.12). Both crossbites and scissors bites can occur unilaterally or bilaterally. If dento-alveolar compensation is present to a marked degree and yet there is still a crossbite or scissors bite, the potential for orthodontic correction is limited.

2.1.2 Soft tissues

The role of the soft tissues in the aetiology of malocclusion is related to both their form and function. In order to understand how these factors operate in producing a malocclusion, it is necessary to understand normal soft tissue form and function. Generally the teeth are considered to adopt a position of balance, between forces applied by the tongue on one side and those applied by the

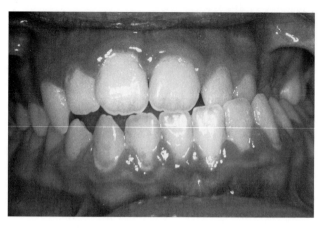

Fig. 2.11   A unilateral crossbite of the maxillary teeth involving the upper left lateral incisor to the left second premolar.

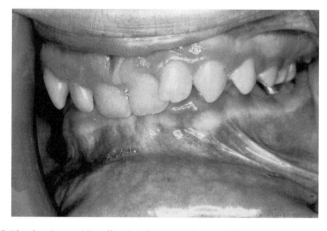

Fig. 2.12   A scissors bite affecting the premolars and first molar on the left.

lips and cheeks on the other. In reality this is an oversimplification, as basic research demonstrates that the loads applied to the buccal and lingual surfaces of teeth are often unequal.[3] However, it is a useful foundation for understanding tooth position.

Normally, the lips are just in contact at rest, with the lower lip covering the incisal third of the upper incisors. During swallowing, the lip to lip anterior oral seal is complete and the tip of the tongue lies just to the palatal of the upper incisors. As swallowing continues the tongue is raised against the hard and then soft palate, and the bolus of food is moved into the pharynx.

A normal class I incisor relationship is thus found with:

(1) lips that are competent at rest as described;
(2) lips which act to form a lip to lip anterior seal with minimal muscular effort; and
(3) a normal tongue behaviour during swallowing.

Tooth position, particularly in the labial segments, will be affected by alterations in the normal soft tissue morphology and behaviour. This is considered in the following sections.

Competent lips with a lip to lip anterior oral seal

Lower lip line and lip competence

Although the lips may be competent, and hence meet at rest with minimal muscular effort, their effect on the labial segment teeth can be modified according to where the lower lip lies in relation to the crowns of the upper incisor teeth. The lower lip covering the incisal third of the crown is important in producing and, in the case of orthodontically treated cases, maintaining a class I incisor relationship. If the lower lip line is very high on the crowns of the upper incisors it may cause all four incisor teeth to be retroclined, creating a class II division 2 incisor relationship (Fig. 2.13). When a high lip position is present during eruption of the permanent incisors it has been noted that the incisors in such patients are often slightly dilacerated in a palatal direction.[4] If the lower lip line is still high and only covers the upper central incisor crowns to a large degree, but does not cover the incisal third of the upper lateral incisors, then the former teeth will be retroclined. The lateral incisors, which are not controlled by the lower lip, will instead be proclined (Fig. 2.14). This will produce the typical appearance of a class II division 2 incisor relationship.

In a case where the lip line is low, such that none of the incisors have their incisal third of the crown covered by the lower lip, the upper incisors will be proclined, producing a class II division 1 incisor relationship.

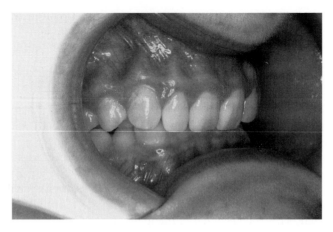

Fig. 2.13   A class II division 2 incisor relationship in which all four upper incisors are retroclined due to the action of the lower lip.

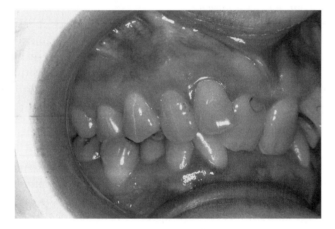

Fig. 2.14   A class II division 2 incisor relationship in which the upper central incisors have been retroclined by the action of the lower lip. The upper lateral incisors are outside lower lip control and as a consequence are proclined, mesially angulated, and mesiolabially rotated.

The examples used to describe the relationship between lip competence, lower lip line, and incisor position are perhaps oversimplifying the true situation, as other factors such as muscle tone and activity of the lips will also have an affect and will be discussed.

Strap like lips

In this case the lips are usually competent and the patien
to lip anterior oral seal. However, there is a great deal of activity in
the circum-oral musculature, which, in association with what is
often a high lower lip line, may cause both the upper and lower
labial segment teeth to be retroclined. This retroclination is known
as bimaxillary retroclination and the incisor relationship in such
cases is usually a severe class II division 2.

Flaccid or full and everted lips

In some patients, mainly as an ethnic characteristic, the circum-
oral musculature appears to have little activity in function. The lips
are usually competent and display a large amount of vermilion
border. Such lips exert little pressure on the labial segment teeth
and as a result the tongue is free to procline the teeth, moulding
them against the inside of the lips. Classically these patients have
proclined upper and lower labial segments, known as bimaxillary
proclination. Although the overjet may be slightly increased, the
incisors may still be in a Class I incisor relationship and the interincisal angle is decreased (Fig. 2.15(a)) or the overjet may be
reduced, creating a class III incisor relationship (Fig. 2.15(b)).

Incompetent lips with an adaptive anterior oral seal

A patient may be unable to obtain a lip to lip anterior oral seal for
a number of reasons. These might include:

- short lips
- a retrognathic mandible
- an increased anterior lower facial height
- prominent upper incisors.

Sometimes a lip to lip anterior oral seal can still be achieved in
spite of the aforementioned reasons. For example, in the case of a
retrognathic mandible or proclined upper incisors, the patient may
posture the mandible forwards to create a lip to lip seal. However, if
the lower lip does not cover the incisal third of the upper incisors at
rest the upper incisors will be proclined. If in such cases the patient
is unable to posture the mandible anteriorly to achieve an anterior
oral seal, then an adaptive anterior oral seal, or adaptive swallowing pattern must be used. These will be discussed in turn.

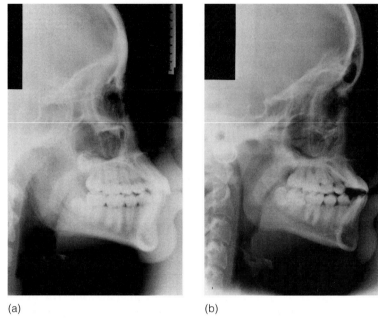

(a)   (b)

Fig. 2.15 Bimaxillary proclination and (a) a class I incisor relationship, (b) a class III incisor relationship.

Tongue to lower lip adaptive swallow
In this instance an anterior oral seal is created when the tip of the tongue moves forwards to meet the lower lip. This is commonly seen in a class II division 1 incisor relationship (see later under Classification), and classically the overbite is increased but just incomplete as a result (Fig. 2.16). The overbite is prevented from becoming complete to either the upper incisors, or as is more usual, to the palatal gingivae, by the interposition of the tongue on swallowing. The separation between the lower incisor edges and the opposing teeth or soft tissues when the patient is in centric occlusion is usually in the region of 1–2 mm. Not only might the upper incisors be proclined as a result of the lack of control by the lower lip, but this may be further compounded by the action of the tongue meeting the lower lip. At the same time, the lower incisors may also be retroclined. As with any adaptive anterior oral seal, on correction of the malocclusion, it is anticipated that soft tissue behaviour will become normal and the treated occlusion remain stable. This will not be the case if the lips are unable to become competent, for

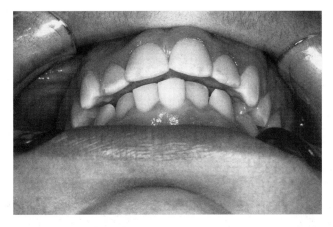

Fig. 2.16 An increased but just incomplete overbite. This is indicative of a tongue to lower lip adaptive anterior oral seal in this class II division 1 incisor relationship.

example in the case of short lips, or a very increased anterior lower facial height. Sometimes a tongue to lower lip adaptive anterior oral seal is seen in combination with a persistent thumb sucking habit. The occlusal features created by the habit, particularly the proclined upper incisors, retroclined lower incisors, and asymmetric anterior open bite, may be perpetuated by the adaptive anterior oral seal, even after cessation of the habit. However, once the occlusal features are corrected, the adaptive anterior oral seal is usually lost and replaced by a normal lip to lip anterior oral seal.

Lower lip to palate
This will occur in similar instances to the tongue to lower lip swallow, only the lower lip contacts the palate during swallowing. As a result, the tongue will not prevent the overbite from becoming increased and complete, usually to the palate or palatal gingivae (Fig. 2.17). The proclination and possible retroclination of the lower incisors will be similar.

Tongue to upper lip adaptive swallow
This can be seen in subjects with a prognathic mandible and where a lip to lip anterior oral seal cannot be achieved. In such cases, the upper incisors may be proclined as a result of the lack of control from the lower lip.

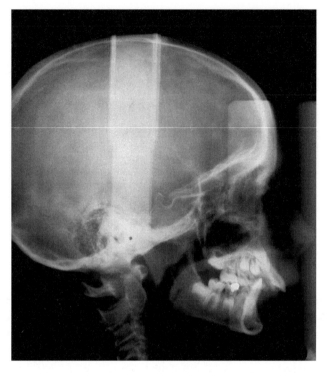

Fig. 2.17 A lateral skull radiograph showing a deep and complete overbite to the palatal gingivae. The overjet or horizontal overlap of the incisors illustrated in this lateral skull radiograph is partly due to the skeletal pattern, and partly to the proclination of the upper incisors.

Atypical swallowing behaviour or 'endogenous' tongue thrust

Rarely, the tongue is thrust quite forcibly forwards against the palatal surface of the upper incisors and indeed between the upper and lower incisors during swallowing. This can lead to the following features being seen:

(1) proclination of both upper and lower labial segments, often with spacing;

(2) a symmetrical incomplete or anterior open bite (Fig. 2.18);

(3) a reverse curve of Spee in the lower arch;

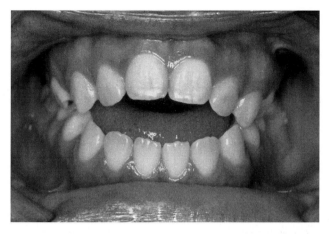

Fig. 2.18 A symmetrical anterior open bite as a consequence of an endogenous tongue thrust. The patient also had a pronounced interdental lisp.

(4) a crenulated border to the tongue as a result of the tongue being continually and forcibly pushed against the lingual surfaces of the teeth;

(5) an interdental lisp;

(6) excessive circum-oral contraction during swallowing.

The first three points are occlusal features. The latter three features may assist in the diagnosis of a tongue thrust but are not exclusive to this condition. It is, however, essential to understand that the presence of a lisp is a reflection of tongue behaviour. It is not a result of a malocclusion *per se*.

It is obviously important to recognize a primary atypical swallowing behaviour before beginning orthodontic treatment. This is because such tongue activity will not adapt to a change in the position of the upper incisors following treatment and relapse will inevitably occur. The presence of an endogenous tongue thrust is said to reflect a primitive swallowing pattern, present from birth. The only reliable method of diagnosing a tongue thrust is to treat the malocclusion and see whether or not relapse occurs. For this reason, any treatment must not compromise the patient's dental health should relapse occur (i.e. consider non-extraction treatment only), and fully informed consent must be obtained, preferably written.

Others

Large tongue

It is difficult to quantify what constitutes a large tongue. However, in many conditions, including Down's syndrome, the patient can have a large and prominent tongue which can lead to proclination of both the upper and lower incisors, along with spacing and a reduced overbite.

Airway considerations

One feature of normal anatomy of the soft tissues often commented upon, and in some cases removed, are the adenoids. It is hypothesized that enlargement of the adenoids blocks normal nasal airflow and as a consequence most breathing is through the mouth, the route of least resistance. In order to accommodate the increased oral airflow the head tends to be tipped back and the mandible drops down, creating a larger freeway space.[5] The typical occlusal effects created include a narrow upper arch, bilateral posterior crossbites, proclined upper incisors, and retroclined lower incisors.

The usual method of assessing the adenoids is by radiographic examination of the lateral skull. At present, however, this subject is controversial and should be considered only by supra-specialist care.

2.1.3 Dento-alveolar factors

These are sometimes referred to as local factors due to their often localized effects on the occlusion. Skeletal malrelationships and soft tissue patterns on the other hand can have a more widespread effect and are commonly referred to as general factors in the aetiology of malocclusion.

Dento-alveolar factors are considered in detail in the following sections.

Anomalies in the number of teeth

Developmentally absent teeth

It is unusual for there to be developmental anomalies in the number of teeth within the deciduous dentition. Missing and extra teeth are most frequently found in the permanent dentition.

The third permanent molars are the most common developmentally absent teeth but are rarely a cause of malocclusion (see

Chapter 9). Developmentally absent second premolars or upper lateral incisors (Fig. 2.19) on the other hand may be implicated in the aetiology of malocclusion and are found to be absent in approximately 5 per cent of children.[6] Their absence can clearly be of major orthodontic significance with a decision commonly having to be made whether to close the resulting space or to reopen or relocate the space prior to replacing the missing tooth or teeth (by implant, fixed or removable prosthesis, or transplant). Since these teeth are commonly missing (Fig. 2.20), it is essential to ascertain their presence, particularly the second premolars, before extracting other teeth for the relief of crowding.

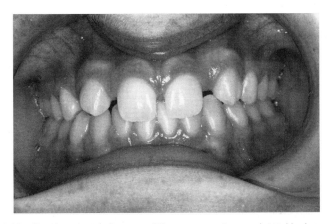

Fig. 2.19   Developmental absence of the permanent upper lateral incisors.

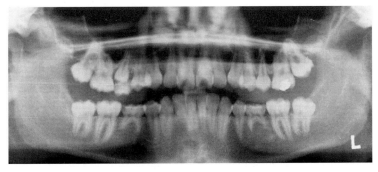

Fig. 2.20   A dental panoramic tomogram (DPT) illustrating developmental absence of lower second premolars.

Lower central incisors are occasionally developmentally absent. Other teeth such as permanent canines, first permanent molars, and upper central incisors are rarely absent.

Early loss of deciduous teeth
The effects of early loss of a deciduous tooth on the occlusion will vary greatly and depend in part on:

- the tooth lost
- age of loss
- tooth arch disproportion (i.e. crowding/spacing)
- intercuspation.

Each of these aspects will now be considered in detail.

The tooth lost   The early loss of a deciduous incisor on its own has little effect on the development of malocclusion. As the effects on the developing dentition are minimal, there is generally no need for any supporting orthodontic treatment such as orthodontic appliances, or balancing or compensating extractions (see Chapter 10). However, trauma may affect the developing occlusion either indirectly via apical pathology or as a direct result of trauma to the deciduous incisors. If the deciduous incisor is intruded as a result of trauma, it can lead to dilaceration of the unerupted permanent successor (Fig. 2.21). This may prevent eruption of the latter tooth, or at least prevent its complete orthodontic realignment into the arch. A dilaceration can occur in either a facial or palatal direction and the determinants of eruption, and/or orthodontic realignment, are principally the site and severity of the dilaceration. If a deciduous incisor is traumatized and undergoes pulpal death, subsequent periapical infection can affect the delicate tissues responsible for crown formation of the permanent successor. This can result in the development of an unsightly area of hypoplastic enamel on the labial surface of the permanent incisor tooth as a consequence of the developmental relationship of the two teeth. Alternatively, if a periapical granuloma and, possibly later, a periapical cyst should develop at the apex of the deciduous incisor, it can prevent the eruption of the permanent successor. In some cases, the cyst not only markedly displaces the permanent successor, but also affects the position of adjacent teeth. The lack of any likely long-term effects on the developing permanent dentition

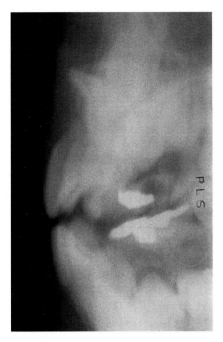

Fig. 2.21   Radiograph showing a dilacerated upper central incisor.

should prompt elective loss of a deciduous incisor with any such associated pathology.

The major effect of early loss of the deciduous canines is to improve the alignment of crowded permanent incisors. If the loss is unilateral (sometimes a deciduous canine will be exfoliated due to resorption of its root by a crowded permanent lateral incisor) the midline will shift to the side of loss and produce an asymmetry in the presence of crowding. For this reason, it is wise to balance the loss of one deciduous canine with the extraction of the other deciduous canine in the same arch.

Incisor crowding in the permanent dentition may also be relieved temporarily by the early loss of first deciduous molars. As in the case of the deciduous canine, unilateral loss of a first deciduous molar can produce a shift of the centreline towards the extraction site. Although there will also be some space loss due to mesial movement of the posterior teeth on the same side, balancing extractions of first deciduous molars should be practised to prevent the development of a dental asymmetry. Alternatively, the loss of a first deciduous molar can be balanced by the loss of the deciduous canine on the opposite side of the same arch.

The primary effect of early loss of a second deciduous molar is to allow the first permanent molar to drift mesially (Fig. 2.22) and encroach on the space reserved for the premolar teeth. In extreme cases the second premolar eventually becomes totally excluded from the arch. There is little effect on the centreline and therefore a balancing extraction of the second deciduous molar on the opposite side of the same arch should not be undertaken.

Age at loss   Clearly, the earlier the deciduous tooth is lost the more pronounced the effects will be. If the tooth in question is close to the normal age at which exfoliation will occur then early loss will have minimal effects on the developing occlusion. For example, if a patient attends at age 12 with a carious second deciduous molar requiring extraction, provided the permanent successor is present, extraction will have little or no effect when compared with loss of the same tooth at age 5.

Tooth arch disproportion (i.e. crowding and spacing)   In spaced arches the early loss of deciduous teeth will have little, if any, effect. In contrast, where there is crowding or potential crowding, the effect will be more pronounced. The early loss of a deciduous tooth does

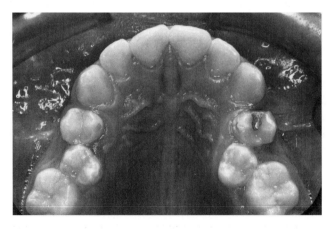

Fig. 2.22   An occlusal photograph showing that the upper second premolar has been excluded from the arch by mesial movement of the first permanent molar as a result of early loss of the upper second deciduous molar.

not create crowding, but merely serves to relocate it within the permanent dentition. This does not mean that early loss of deciduous teeth is unimportant. Subsequent treatment of crowding in the permanent dentition may be more difficult following the uncontrolled drift of permanent teeth.

Intercuspation   Good intercuspation of the first permanent molars may reduce space loss if there has been early loss of a deciduous tooth in only one arch, but not if a tooth has also been lost on the same side in the opposing arch.

Retained deciduous teeth   A deciduous tooth is often retained beyond its normal time of shedding when the permanent successor is absent or misplaced. For example, an upper deciduous canine may be retained when the permanent canine is ectopically placed, most commonly palatally. However, in some circumstances, retention of a deciduous tooth will in itself prevent eruption of the permanent successor, or result in its deflection from its normal path of eruption. If a lower deciduous incisor root is not resorbed by its permanent successor, the permanent incisor will be deflected lingually. The process of shedding of a deciduous tooth is known to be a dynamic one in which the root undergoes resorption and repair at differing rates. Sometimes repair occurs at a greater rate than does resorption and the tooth becomes ankylosed to the alveolar bone. In the growing child, the surrounding teeth and their supporting alveolar bone will continue to grow in an occlusal direction, so that the ankylosed tooth is left behind and appears to submerge (Fig. 2.23). A submerging deciduous molar may be associated with the absence of a permanent successor, but if the premolar is present it will be prevented from erupting. Usually such ankylosis resolves spontaneously, the deciduous tooth re-emerges, and is eventually shed. However, if a deciduous molar submerges by more than 2–3 mm, such that its occlusal surface appears to be below the normal contact points of the adjacent teeth, it should either have its occlusal surface height restored along with its proximal contacts,[7] or it should be extracted. In the former case, provided the permanent successor continues to erupt normally, the deciduous tooth will eventually be exfoliated.

Occasionally a deciduous tooth is retained as a result of infection. If an area of chronic infection develops at the apex of a deciduous tooth it may be retained and prevent the eruption of the permanent successor.

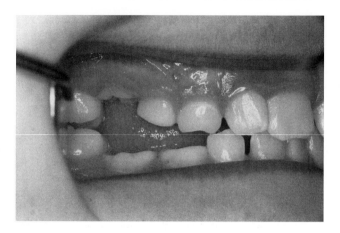

Fig. 2.23 A buccal view showing submergence of the first and second decidu-ous molars as a consequence of ankylosis. The submergence has gone beyond the interproximal contacts.

Unscheduled loss of permanent teeth

Loss of permanent teeth as a result of trauma, caries, or periodontal disease may be detrimental to the occlusion. In general, the effect on the occlusion will depend upon a number of factors, some of which are seen with early loss of deciduous teeth, and some of which are not. Some of these factors are listed below.

1. The degree of crowding. If there is no crowding then the effect on the remaining teeth in the same arch will be minimal. However, in the opposing arch there may be over-eruption of the opposing tooth.

2. The age at tooth loss. Loss of a permanent tooth before full development of the permanent dentition may result in adjacent teeth erupting into the space created. For example, loss of an upper lateral incisor prior to the eruption of the permanent canine can result in the canine erupting into the site of the lateral incisor, pro-vided space loss has not occurred due to drifting of adjacent teeth. The deciduous canine may also be retained as a result, since its root will not be resorbed by the permanent canine. Early loss of the first permanent molars can have a similar effect on the second permanent molars (see later).

3. The site of tooth loss. If there is crowding within the arch then the loss of a permanent tooth will have a greater effect if it is close to the site of crowding. For instance, the loss of an upper lateral incisor when there is labial segment crowding may lead to rapid space loss. The adjacent teeth will tip into the extraction site, resulting in a marked shift in the upper centreline. In the same case, loss of an upper second permanent molar is likely to have little effect, as the site of tooth loss is some way away from the principal site of crowding. It may, however, permit the eruption into function of an upper third permanent molar, which would not have been possible following loss of the incisor tooth.

4. The angulation of adjacent teeth. If the long axes of these teeth are angulated away from an extraction site, then space loss may be rapid as they move to a normal angulation into the space created. As a result, the final angulations of the adjacent teeth, once the space has closed, may be perfectly acceptable, as might the resulting contact between the teeth. If, however, the adjacent teeth are initially angulated towards the extraction site, space loss may not be so rapid or as complete. This might result in residual space remaining and adjacent teeth markedly tipped into the extraction site.

5. Interdigitation of adjacent teeth. If the teeth adjacent to the extraction site interdigitate well with the opposing teeth, this may prevent their movement into the extraction site.

The first molars are the permanent teeth most frequently lost as a result of caries.[8] Their loss can result in a major derangement of the occlusion, especially when extracted after the age of 10 years. Space closure, particularly in the lower arch, will be unsatisfactory, with adjacent teeth tilting into the extraction site. If the extractions are performed between the ages of 8 and 10 years, that is, prior to root formation of the second permanent molars, these latter teeth will usually erupt further mesially and a reasonable approximal contact may be achieved between the second permanent molar and the second premolars (Fig. 2.24).

The effect of late extraction of maxillary first molars is less marked. In these cases the mesial position of the second molar root apices, compared with the crown, ensures that tipping of this tooth will lead to a suitable contact point with the maxillary second premolar.

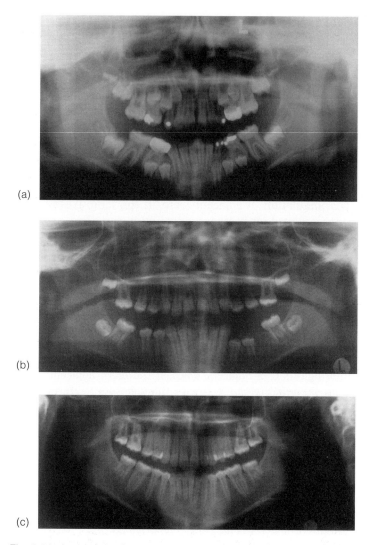

(a)

(b)

(c)

Fig. 2.24 Loss of the first permanent molars between the ages of 8 and 10 years can allow the second molars to erupt into a good position. This shows a series of three radiographs of a patient with a history of irregular attendance. Initially (a) the patient was seen at age 7 – note the caries present at this stage. The next attendance was at age $9\frac{1}{2}$ for acute pulpitic problems. A radiograph six months later (b) shows clearly the treatment undertaken. The patient at age 19 has been fortunate, with the resulting occlusion (c) being acceptable to both patient and practitioner.

Extra teeth

Additional teeth prior to the normal development of the deciduous dentition are discussed elsewhere (Chapter 1). It is rare to find extra teeth in the deciduous dentition. Extra teeth within the permanent dentition may resemble teeth of the normal series, in which case they are referred to as supplemental teeth, or they may be different from the normal series in which case they are known as supernumerary teeth.

A supernumerary tooth commonly found close to the midline in the upper arch is known as a mesiodens (Fig. 2.25). These teeth are usually peg-shaped and may or may not erupt. Although they may displace the permanent central incisors from their normal path of eruption, they do not prevent the eruption of these teeth.

Tuberculate supernumeraries, or tuberculate odontomes as they are sometimes known, not only fail to erupt, but also prevent the eruption of the upper central incisor (Fig. 2.26). Whenever a tooth demonstrates delayed eruption relative to the rest of the developing occlusion, or if a tooth is displaced from its normal path of eruption, an intra-oral radiograph should be taken. A useful guide in the determination of delayed eruption is to look for asymmetry of development within the same arch. If, for example, one of the upper central incisor crowns has been visible in the

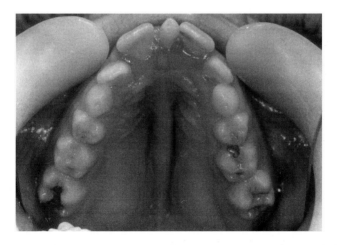

Fig. 2.25 A photograph showing a midline supernumerary tooth or mesiodens between the upper central incisors.

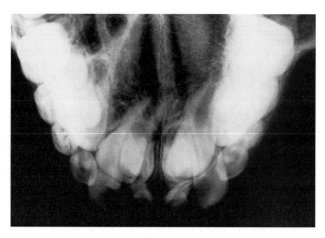

Fig. 2.26   An upper standard maxillary occlusal radiograph showing a tuberculate supernumerary overlying the cingulum of each of the unerupted upper central incisors.

mouth for 6–9 months and yet the contralateral tooth is still only palpable under the mucosa, the situation should be investigated further, usually radiographically.

In the case of the maxillary central incisors a nasal occlusal (upper standard maxillary occlusal) view should be obtained. Using this film it will be possible to differentiate a mesiodens from a tuberculate supernumerary tooth. The former is usually seen lying between the roots of the maxillary central incisors, while the tuberculate supernumerary tooth is seen overlying the cingulum plateau of the permanent central incisor. Not infrequently two tuberculate supernumerary teeth are seen, one overlying each upper central incisor. Where necessary the extra tooth should be extracted. Orthodontic treatment may also be required to align the central incisors, or to maintain the space whilst awaiting their eruption. Sometimes, a mesiodens is found by chance on a radiograph and will have no effect on the occlusion. Provided it remains unerupted and high above the roots of the incisors it can be left in position. If it is likely to interfere with orthodontic treatment, due to its close proximity to the roots of the upper central incisors, it will have to be removed.

Extra teeth may also be found elsewhere in the mouth, usually in the upper lateral, lower incisor, and lower premolar regions.

These are often supplemental teeth, being indistinguishable from teeth of the normal series. If crowding is present, then the tooth furthest from the line of the arch is usually extracted (Fig. 2.27). This decision may be modified according to the condition of the teeth and supporting tissues. For example, a tooth with caries, a history of trauma, or marked gingival recession, all of which might affect long-term prognosis, may make it the tooth of choice for extraction.

Occasionally the presence of an erupted supplemental tooth has little effect on the occlusion, which would otherwise have been spaced. Obviously in this situation the tooth should be accepted.

Dento-alveolar disproportion – crowding/spacing

This is where the mesiodistal widths of the teeth are dissimilar to the length of the alveolus. As a result there may be generalized spacing or generalized crowding throughout the arch. Although the mismatch between the tooth sizes and the alveolus may be generalized, the spacing or crowding may instead be localized within the arch. In addition, there may be little correlation between the mesiodistal widths of the upper and the lower arch teeth. This can

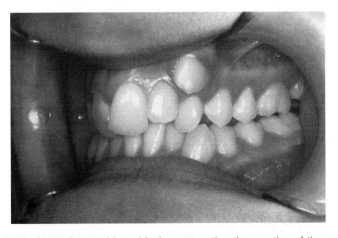

Fig. 2.27 A supplemental lateral incisor preventing the eruption of the upper permanent canine. Extraction of the lateral incisor furthest from the correct position in the arch will relieve the crowding present and permit the eruption of the canine tooth.

result in the buccal segment teeth not being fully interdigitated, or there being crowding in just one arch whilst the opposing arch teeth are well aligned. Often the discrepancy in tooth size between the upper and lower arches is very subtle and indeed may only become evident at the end of a course of orthodontic treatment when opposing teeth do not fully interdigitate.

Anomalies in tooth form

Although, anomalies in tooth form can include dento-alveolar disproportion, this terminology is usually reserved for specific localized abnormalities of form. Such abnormalities include excessively large teeth (megadont) (Fig. 2.28) and small teeth (e.g. peg-shaped upper lateral incisors), both of which will have an obvious effect on the occlusion via increased crowding or spacing within the arch.

Not infrequently, in association with peg-shaped lateral incisors, there is a pronounced pit close to the incisal edge of the tooth. In extreme cases this pit is very deep and radiographically can be seen as a deep invagination of the crown passing down into the pulp. Such a tooth is known as an invaginated odontome or 'dens in dente' (tooth within a tooth). Not only is this deep invaginated pit prone to caries, but the enamel and dentine overlying the pulp, within the pit, is very thin. A carious lesion can

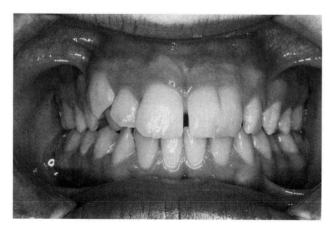

Fig. 2.28 A megadont upper central incisor.

therefore progress quickly towards the pulp. Subsequent root treatment is difficult and often unsatisfactory, and extraction is often the only sensible long term treatment option. This will have obvious consequences for the occlusion. For this reason invaginated odontomes should be fissure sealed soon after eruption if the tooth is to be retained.

Other abnormalities of form such as accessory cusps (e.g. talon cusps) or accessory ridges (Fig. 2.29) may not have any effect mesiodistally within the arch, unlike excessively large or small teeth, but may instead prevent correct interocclusal relationships between the upper and lower arch teeth vertically or labiolingually. Anomalies in tooth form due to environmental rather than genetic effects may also be implicated in the aetiology of malocclusion. For example, dilacerated teeth often develop as a result of traumatic injury, and depending on the site and severity of the dilaceration, the tooth may or may not erupt. If it does erupt, the dilaceration may preclude either normal eruption or subsequent alignment into the arch using an orthodontic appliance (see 'Early loss of deciduous teeth').

Anomalies in tooth position

Any tooth may develop in an abnormal position, although this is most commonly seen with upper permanent canines and lower

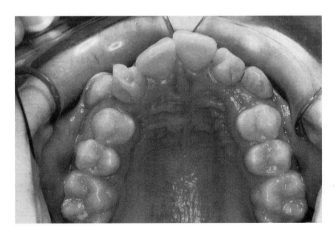

Fig. 2.29   Accessory ridges on upper lateral incisor teeth.

third permanent molars. Other anomalies of position reflecting abnormal development of the teeth include inversions (Fig. 2.30), transpositions (e.g. the positions of the canine and second premolar or lateral incisor may be reversed; Fig. 2.31), and severe rotations (Fig. 2.32).

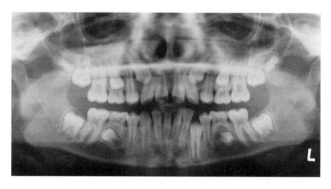

Fig. 2.30 A DPT radiograph showing an inverted mandibular left premolar, in which case extraction of the deciduous teeth will not resolve the problem.

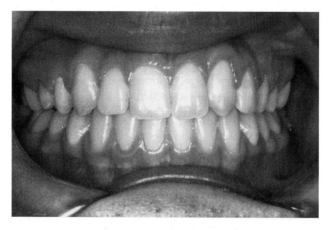

Fig. 2.31 Transposition of the upper left permanent canine and lateral incisor in an otherwise satisfactory occlusion. The patient was unaware of the problem and so no orthodontic treatment was undertaken.

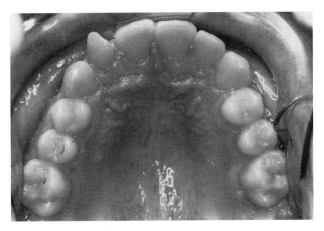

Fig. 2.32   A severely rotated upper right lateral incisor, rotated through 90°.

Abnormal frenum

In the infant the upper labial frenum extends from the inner surface of the lip to the palatine papilla. As the teeth erupt, this continuity is lost and the frenum becomes attached to the labial surface of the alveolar process. Occasionally, the frenum will persist and be associated with a median diastema. In such cases the palatine papilla will blanch if the lip is pulled forwards. It should be remembered that a median diastema prior to the eruption of the permanent canines and during the mixed dentition is a normal finding. In the majority of cases this diastema will close spontaneously upon eruption of the permanent canines. However, if the frenum is thick and fleshy it may prevent this closure. In these unusual cases, a frenectomy may be indicated, particularly if the frenum is large and pendulous and is preventing a patient from maintaining a good standard of oral hygiene around the adjacent upper central incisors (Fig. 2.33). However, frenectomy alone is unlikely to have much of an effect in terms of spontaneous space closure and appliance therapy is usually required to close the diastema.

Another frenum, and one which is rarely implicated in the aetiology of malocclusion, is the lingual frenum. It can very occasionally be related to a median diastema in the lower arch. However, the indications for its removal, both from the point of view of aesthetics and function, are very limited.

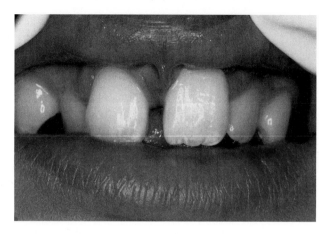

Fig. 2.33 A large fleshy upper labial frenum tethering the upper lip.

Pathology

Chronic periodontitis
Periodontal tissue breakdown has been linked with drifting of the maxillary labial segments in older patients and is reported to occur as a consequence of disruption in the principal collagen fibres of the periodontium. Most of the inflammation and bone loss which occurs does so on the palatal aspect of these teeth. The upper incisors therefore tend to drift labially away from the site of inflammation, becoming proclined and spaced. Possible theories as to why the incisors drift include:

(1) the presence of a greater degree of disease on the palatal aspect of the teeth;
(2) production of granulation tissue palatally;
(3) disruption of the restraining periodontal ligament fibres;
(4) a reduction in supportive root length (i.e. that still supported by the periodontium within the alveolar bone).

Juvenile periodontitis
A less common form of periodontal disease is juvenile periodontitis, where rapid bone loss around the roots of the first permanent molars and central incisors can seriously affect the long term prognosis of these teeth. While a number of more recent techniques are

being advocated for the treatment of this condition, none as yet can replace the lost bone. It is also difficult to predict the effect this localized bone loss has on teeth which are subsequently to be moved into the area since there is no clear evidence as to the formation of an alveolus commensurate with health.

Cysts/tumours
Cysts of inflammatory and developmental origin can not only prevent the eruption of teeth but also displace them from their normal eruptive path (Fig. 2.34). An example of a cyst of inflammatory origin is a periapical cyst in a deciduous incisor, and an example of a developmental cyst is a dentigerous cyst on the crown of a permanent tooth. Both may prevent permanent tooth eruption. Rarely, tumours such as an adenomatoid odontogenic tumour can prevent the eruption of a permanent tooth.

2.1.4 Habits

The habits of orthodontic significance are thumb- and finger sucking. The following discussion refers to thumb sucking but the comments apply equally to finger sucking.

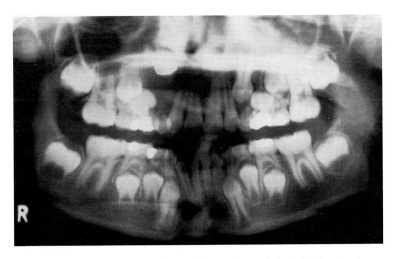

Fig. 2.34 A cyst of developmental or inflammatory origin deflecting the upper right maxillary canine tooth from its normal path of eruption.

Thumb sucking does not always have an effect on the occlusion. The magnitude of any effect will depend on the force applied to the teeth, and also the frequency and duration of the habit. Thumb sucking is very common in young infants and may be regarded as normal behaviour. If the habit persists into the deciduous dentition a malocclusion may be produced, but this is not usually considered to be of long term orthodontic significance. Treatment to stop the habit is not indicated since the child may depend greatly on the habit for comfort and support. The effects on the deciduous occlusion may include:

(1) proclination of the upper incisors;

(2) retroclination of the lower incisors;

(3) reduction of the overbite which will be incomplete and often asymmetric;

(4) narrowing of the upper arch to match the width of the lower;

(5) development of a unilateral crossbite with a displacement.

The mechanism of upper incisor proclination and lower incisor retroclination is fairly obvious, as is the reduced overbite or asymmetric anterior open bite. The maxillary arch narrowing with crossbite formation occurs due to the thumb being held against the palate. The tongue is forced to move down towards the floor of the mouth. As the tongue occupies more space than the thumb, and the thumb is sucked with the teeth apart, the tongue is able to maintain the lower arch width. The thumb, however, will not be able to resist the forces applied to the upper buccal segment teeth from the cheeks during sucking. As a result, the upper arch narrows whilst the lower arch width remains the same. Once the maxillary and mandibular arch widths become equal, the patient's teeth will occlude in a cusp to cusp relationship. The mandible must therefore displace to one side on closing into centric occlusion so that the buccal segment teeth can move from a cusp to cusp relationship into a position of maximum intercuspation. Therefore the patient has a unilateral crossbite with a mandibular displacement on closing into centric occlusion (see Chapter 6). It should be noted that unless there is extensive occlusal wear of the deciduous teeth, this displacement will persist into the mixed dentition so that the crossbite and displacement are perpetuated. Nevertheless, treatment is better left until the child is ready to give up the habit, especially if social factors play a part in the initiation of the habit.

The effects of thumb sucking on the permanent dentition are the same as in the deciduous dentition (Fig. 2.35). By the age of 10 years most children are ready to give up the habit and many do so spontaneously. However, if encouragement is not sufficient, a simple removable reminder plate will often be successful. Use of nail biting solutions and sticking plasters have variable rates of success. A more successful method can be to break the seal produced during the habit and a common way of doing this is with a glove. Following cessation of the habit the incisor relationship may improve spontaneously. If it does not, appliance treatment will be necessary. A unilateral crossbite with an associated lateral displacement of the mandible will not resolve without appliance therapy.

Summary of factors involved in the aetiology of malocclusion

There are four main aetiological factors involved in the development of malocclusion and in any single case, one or more of them may be implicated in its aetiology. Certainly the four factors are often closely related. For example, an increased overjet (the horizontal overlap of the incisors) might be determined by skeletal pattern and the inclination of the upper incisors (see Fig. 2.17) and both in turn may modify what in other cases might be the principal aetiological agent, namely soft tissue behaviour. If an increased overjet is due to a digit sucking habit, then any adaptive swallow which occurs as a consequence can maintain the increased overjet, even after cessation of the habit. Other features of a malocclusion can similarly be used to demonstrate how the principal aetiological agents might operate. Overbite (the vertical overlap of the incisors) will be dependent on the same factors, as listed below:

(1) skeletal pattern – vertical and anteroposterior;
(2) soft tissues (e.g. adaptive swallowing behaviour);
(3) habits;
(4) dento-alveolar factors (e.g. the interincisal angle, see later, and the form of the palatal surfaces of the upper incisors).

It is because the aetiology of malocclusion is multifactorial that a thorough and systematic approach to examination and diagnosis of the orthodontic patient must be performed. It is easy to plan a treatment around correction of the most obvious aspects of the malocclusion and to miss other factors, which might have a significant effect on the complexity, outcome, and long term stability of any treatment.

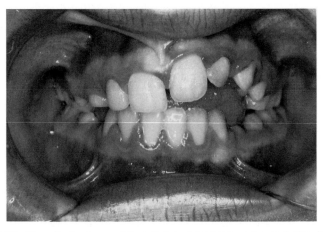

Fig. 2.35   The effects of a persistent digit sucking habit on the occlusion. Notice the characteristic asymmetry of the open bite created.

2.2 CLASSIFICATION OF MALOCCLUSION

Occlusal and facial patterns vary widely and in many circumstances it is convenient to categorize them into a small number of groups. The objective of any system of classification is to gather together cases with similar features or with a common aetiology. Individuals within a class should ideally resemble one another more closely in the relevant features than individuals in other classes. However, as with many biological attributes, there is a spectrum of continuous variation and the division between classes is arbitrary. This makes the designation of borderline cases difficult. Methods of classifying malocclusions and facial patterns have been developed intuitively, and when modern statistical techniques are used to investigate the most efficient systems, these generally do not correspond with the time-honoured patterns, which nevertheless persist. However, the importance of classification in everyday clinical practice should not be exaggerated. The classification of a malocclusion cannot constitute a full description, nor is it the basis for the prescription of treatment.

Different methods of classification may be needed for different purposes, and an appropriate method must be adopted for the task in hand. For instance the requirements of clinical categorization differ from those of epidemiology. Angle's classification is the most commonly used in clinical orthodontic practice.[9] However, it would not be suitable for investigating the relationship between dental irregularity and problems such as periodontal disease due to its very character.

2.2.1 Angle's classification

Angle's classification is based on arch relationship in the sagittal plane, derived from the position of the first permanent molars. In normal occlusion the mesiobuccal cusp of the upper first permanent molar occludes with the anterior buccal groove of the lower first permanent molar. In other words, Angle felt that the first molars were always in the same position and that any alteration in the relationship of the upper and lower first permanent molars was a reflection of an underlying skeletal discrepancy. There are three Angle's classes, I, II, and III. These are defined below.

1. Angle's class I: Malocclusions in which there is a normal anteroposterior arch relationship judged by the first permanent molars and where the mesiobuccal cusp of the upper first permanent molar occludes with the anterior buccal groove of the lower first permanent molar (Fig. 2.36).

2. Angle's class II: The lower arch is at least one half cusp width distal to the upper, as judged by the relationship of the first permanent molars. Class II is further divided according to the incisor relationship.

    - Division 1: The upper central incisors are of average inclination or proclined so that there is an increase in overjet (Fig. 2.37).

    - Division 2: The upper central incisors are retroclined. Characteristically, the lateral incisors may be proclined, mesially angulated, and mesiolabially rotated (Fig. 2.37). The overbite is usually increased. The overjet may be average, decreased, or increased but usually by only a small amount.

3. Angle's class III: The lower arch is at least one half a cusp width mesial to the upper, as judged by the relationship of the first permanent molars (Fig. 2.36).

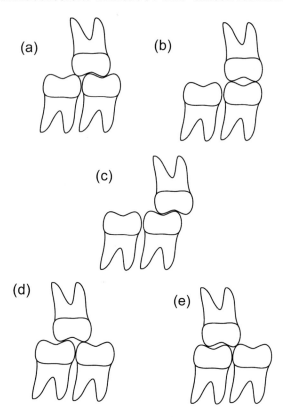

Fig. 2.36 Molar relationships: (a) class I, (b) $\frac{1}{2}$ unit class II, (c) class II, (d) $\frac{1}{2}$ unit class III, (e) class III. Note that it is also possible to describe molar relationships as $\frac{1}{4}$ and $\frac{3}{4}$ unit class II or class III. On the left of the figure are the distal surfaces of the teeth and on the right the mesial surfaces.

This critical reliance on the molar relationship as representing the underlying skeletal pattern is the major shortcoming of Angle's classification. For example, the first permanent molars may be missing or may have drifted following early loss of deciduous teeth and have to be repositioned mentally before classification. Alternatively, the molar relationship may differ between the two sides of the mouth. Whatever the situation the molar relationship is a poor assessment of sagittal skeletal arch relationships. For this reason Angle's description is used for buccal segment relationships and incisor classifications, whilst the skeletal relationship must be assessed and described separately.

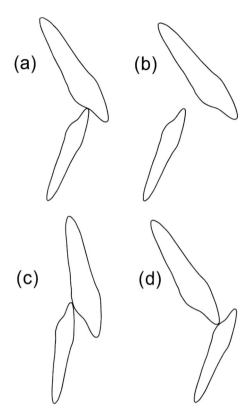

Fig. 2.37   Incisor relationships: (a) class I, (b) class II division 1, (c) class II
division 2, (d) class III.

2.2.2 Current use of incisor classification and definitions

Although Angle's original classification suffered from the miscon-
ception that the skeletal relationship could be determined by the
position of the first permanent molars, many facets of the
classification are still in use today. These include the molar and
incisor classifications. The definitions of incisor relationship have
evolved from specific measurements of the overjet and overbite,
previously expressed as being a 2–4 mm horizontal overlap with a
vertical overlap of one third of the crown of the lower incisors in a
class I incisor relationship. The more formally recorded British
standards (see Glossary) are given.

1. Class I: The lower incisor edges occlude with or lie directly below the cingulum plateau of the upper central incisors. If the overbite is incomplete the lower incisors are repositioned along their long axis until they meet the upper incisors (Fig. 2.37).

2. Class II: The lower incisor edges lie posterior to the cingulum plateau of the upper central incisors. There are two divisions of class II:

   - Division 1: The upper central incisors are of average inclination or are proclined. The overjet is thus increased (Fig. 2.37).

   - Division 2: The upper central incisors are retroclined; the overjet is usually within normal limits but the overbite is often increased (Fig. 2.37).

3. Class III: The lower incisor edges lie anterior to the cingulum plateau of the upper central incisors (Fig. 2.37).

2.2.3 Current use of molar/canine classification and definitions

Angle's description of molar relationships has been superseded by that of Andrews, which forms one of the 'six keys to normal occlusion'.[10] The normal, and hence class I relationship, is defined as being present when the distal surface of the upper first permanent molar distobuccal cusp occludes with the mesiobuccal cusp of the lower second permanent molar. Although this definition of a class I molar relationship is perhaps more accurate, Angle's system of classification of molar relationships is still in common usage. Whatever system is used, if the molar relationship is not a full unit class I, II, or III then fractions of a unit of class II or III are used.

The definitions of canine relationship are as follows.

1. Class I canine relationship – the upper permanent canine occludes in the embrasure between the lower permanent canine and the first premolar.

2. Class II canine relationship – the upper canine occludes a whole tooth width further anteriorly and lies in the embrasure between the lower canine and lateral incisor.

3. Class III canine relationship – the upper canine occludes a whole tooth width further posteriorly than normal and occludes in the embrasure between the lower first and second premolars.

As with molar relationship, where necessary the relationship can be described as a fraction of a unit discrepancy if it is somewhere between class I and either class II or class III. For example, it is possible to have a $\frac{1}{4}$, $\frac{1}{2}$, or $\frac{3}{4}$ unit class II canine relationship (Fig. 2.38).

By describing buccal segment relationships in this manner, including fractions of a unit, the clinician is able to assess potential anchorage requirements in the correction of a malocclusion. For example, a half unit class II buccal segment relationship might indicate the potential need for headgear therapy or extractions alone, whereas a full unit class II would be difficult to correct with

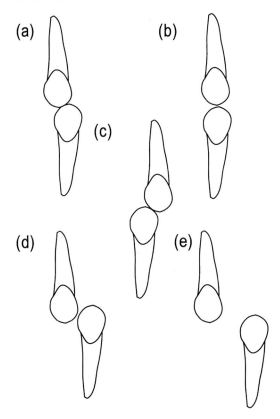

Fig. 2.38 Canine relationships: (a) class I, (b) $\frac{1}{2}$ unit class II, (c) class II, (d) $\frac{1}{2}$ unit class III, (e) class III. Note that it is possible to describe canine relationships as $\frac{1}{4}$ and $\frac{3}{4}$ unit class II or class III. The orientation is as in Fig. 2.36.

standard techniques. Advanced mechanics, including functional appliances, or the skilled use of headgear would be appropriate.

If there is a discrepancy between the assessed molar and canine relationships on one side then the cause of the discrepancy must be sought.

Sometimes it is not possible to assess the buccal segment relationship using the first permanent molars (e.g. if one or more have been extracted). In this case it will be necessary to describe either the premolar or the canine relationship. This is appropriate as the canine teeth are often the cornerstone of treatment. Failure to achieve a class I canine relationship will usually result in a failure to correct the incisor relationship.

2.2.4 Skeletal classification and definitions

Anteroposterior

A class I skeletal pattern is seen when the maxilla is slightly ahead of the mandible. Class II occurs when the mandible appears to be more posterior than this and class III when the mandible appears to be more anterior than the maxilla (see Chapter 4). Skeletal pattern can also be classified using measurements obtained from lateral skull radiographs. In this case the assessment is made using the angle ANB (see p. 173). An ANB angle of 2°–4° denotes a class I skeletal pattern, greater than 4° is class II, and less than 2° is Class III. This will be discussed further in Chapter 8.

Within the class II and class III skeletal categories the severity of the discrepancy can be described further as mild, moderate, or severe, adding further emphasis to the potential mechanism for treatment. This is discussed later in Chapter 4.

Vertical

There is no suitable classification of vertical facial dimensions, although as discussed earlier, facial types can sometimes be divided into anterior and posterior growth rotators. In general terms the face is described as it presents, by noting the vertical facial proportions. The face is conveniently divided into thirds (see Chapter 4) and in particular it is the lower third of the face that is of specific interest in orthodontics. This is usually described as being an average, increased, or decreased anterior lower face height. In addition the facial proportions can also be described in terms of the angle between the mandible and the maxilla and is either normal, increased, or decreased. How this assessment is made is detailed in Chapter 4.

Transverse

Again this is purely descriptive and outlines the extent of any transverse discrepancies. There is no formal classification of transverse discrepancy although any intra-oral effect, such as a crossbite, can usually be classified. These will be discussed in Chapter 5.

2.2.5 Case summary

In describing any case it is helpful to have a one- or two-sentence description of the salient features. A typical case description would be: 'the patient presented with a class II division 1 incisor relationship on a class II skeletal base complicated by a digit sucking habit. The buccal segments are one half unit class II'. In this way the case is visualized mentally when reporting to another clinician.

The order of presentation differs from the order in which the information is gleaned during the examination, in that incisal relationship is presented first, followed by skeletal pattern, and then possible aetiological factors. Although the case summary uses incisal, skeletal, and sometimes buccal segment classifications, it is mainly descriptive and does not constitute a complete classification of the malocclusion.

2.2.6 Other classifications and their purpose

The preceding incisor, canine, molar, and skeletal classifications can be used to describe individual facets of a presenting malocclusion either in detail or as a case summary. However, such descriptive classifications are limited, for example as a measure of the severity of a presenting malocclusion, or how easily it might be treated. They are also of limited value in the determination of cases which would benefit the most from treatment, where treatment services are limited, or in the investigation of the relationships between malocclusion and various aspects of dental health.

In an attempt to overcome these shortcomings several indices of malocclusion have been proposed. None is entirely satisfactory and it is unlikely that any single index will be suitable for all purposes.

Before any index is adopted for use, it should prove to be valid (does it in fact measure what is required?) and reproducible (do observers consistently obtain the same values for a series of test cases?).

Two of the most established indices of malocclusion for prioritizing treatment in other countries with limited care availability are the handicapping malocclusion assessment record (HMAR) and the occlusal index (OI).[11,12] Both perform reasonably well for reproducibility and validity.

The HMAR allocates points for dental irregularities and arch malrelationships, which are multiplied by a weighting factor before the total score is assigned. This can be done from orthodontic models or at a clinical assessment. In the latter case, further points can be allotted for dentofacial deviations such as clefts of the lip and palate, facial asymmetry, and functional disabilities. The assessment is quite rapid and does not require special instruments.

The OI scores dental age, molar relations, overbite, overjet, posterior crossbite, posterior open bite, tooth displacement, midline relations, and missing upper lateral incisors. A number of measurements are involved and the scoring is rather more complicated than for the HMAR, but it is a more reliable method of ranking the severity of malocclusion.

Another index, the PAR (peer assessment rating) index is used mainly to judge the effectiveness of treatment, as it is not a descriptive index. There are two basic types, weighted and unweighted. The main value of the PAR index is that it is performed on study models away from the clinical environment and as such has two advantages. First, it can be performed by non-clinical auxiliary staff and second, the results of treatment can therefore be judged in an unbiased manner. By scoring pre- and post-treatment study models the possible efficacy of orthodontic treatment can be judged although the precision of this index still remains to be defined.[13]

The index of treatment need (IOTN) is another mechanism of prioritizing and thereby classifying malocclusions according to treatment need.[14] This is particularly useful where the resources available for treatment are limited. This index is discussed further in Chapter 7.

Summary of classification of malocclusion

1. Incisor relationship:
    (a) Class I
    (b) Class II
        (i)   Division 1
        (ii) Division 2
    (c) Class III
2. Molar and canine relationships. These can be Class I, II, III, or fractions of a tooth unit of the latter two classes. (A tooth unit is a mesiodistal premolar width.)
3. Sagittal skeletal relationship is also classified into classes I, II, or III with the latter two being further subdivided into mild, moderate, or severe.
4. Vertical skeletal relationships are usually described with respect to the Frankfort–mandibular planes angle and anterior lower facial height rather than classified. However, some faces can be classified as 'high' or 'low' angle faces.
5. Transverse skeletal relationship are described and not classified.

Objectives

Classification

- List all classifications of the incisor relationship and variants
- List the classifications of the buccal segment relationships
- Outline Angle's classification
- List some indices commonly used in orthodontics

REFERENCES

1. Björk, A. (1969). Prediction of mandibular growth rotation. *American Journal of Orthodontics*, **55**, 585–99.
2. Akerly, B. A. (1977). Prosthodontic treatment of traumatic overlap of the anterior teeth. *Journal of Prosthetic Dentistry*, **38**, 26–34.
3. Proffit, W. R., Chastain, B. B., and Norton, L. A. (1969). Linguo-palatal pressure in children. *American Journal of Orthodontics*, **55**, 154–66.

4. Delivanis, H. P. and Kuftinec, M. M. (1980). Variation in the morphology of the maxillary central incisors found in class II division 2 malocclusions. *American Journal of Orthodontics*, **78**, 438–44.
5. Behlfelt, K., Linder-Aronson, S., McWilliam, J. Neander, P., and Laage-Hellman, J. (1990). Craniofacial morphology in children with and without enlarged tonsils. *European Journal of Orthodontics*, **12**, 233–43.
6. Maklin, M., Dummett, C. O., and Weinberg, R. (1979). A study of oligodontia in a sample of New Orleans children. *Journal of Dentistry for Children*, **46**, 478–82.
7. Kurol, J. and Magnusson, B. C. (1984). Infraocclusion of primary molars: a histological study. *Scandinavian Journal of Dental Research*, **92**, 564–76.
8. Office of population censuses and surveys (OPCS) (1994). *Children's dental health in the United Kingdom*. HMSO, London.
9. Angle, E. H. (1899). Classification of malocclusion. *Dental Cosmos*, **41**, 248–64, 350–7.
10. Andrews, L. F. (1972). The six keys to normal occlusion. *American Journal of Orthodontics*, **62**, 296–309.
11. Salzmann, J. A. (1967). Malocclusion severity assessment. *American Journal of Orthodontics*, **53**, 109–19.
12. Summers, C. J. (1971). The occlusal index: a system for identifying and scoring occlusal disorders. *American Journal of Orthodontics*, **59**, 552–67.
13. Shaw, W. C., Richmond, S., O'Brien, K. D., Brook, P., and Stephens, C. D. (1991). Quality control in orthodontics: indices of treatment need and treatment standards. *British Dental Journal*, **170**, 107–12.
14. Brook, P. H. and Shaw, W. C. (1989). The development of an index of orthodontic treatment priority. *European Journal of Orthodontics*, **11**, 309–20.

3

Patient and parent interview

The patient and parent interview serves a number of important functions. To begin with it is likely to be the first experience the patient has of the processes involved in orthodontic treatment. It is also a time when the clinician must obtain information from the patient not only on their orthodontic concerns, but on factors which might have a bearing on any proposed treatment. Specific factors may come to light on questioning the patient about their medical and dental history. Less specific information, including straightforward and obvious domestic issues such as ease of travel for treatment, also needs to be determined. Such information might influence the clinician to modify the complexity of any proposed treatment plan.

Essentially the interview is aimed at assessing the suitability and, in particular, the motivation of both patient and parent towards orthodontic treatment. As such it needs to be conducted in a relaxed but ordered manner. Some clinicians interview patients separately from their parents while others prefer to have the parent in the surgery at the same time. If the parent is present, it is essential to ensure that most of the interview is conducted with the child and not to the child via the parent. In such circumstances it is important that the clinician has command of the interview so the necessary information can be gained in an efficient yet considerate manner.

The typical order of the patient and parent interview is as follows:

(1) presenting complaint
(2) past medical history
(3) past dental history
(4) explanation of possible orthodontic treatment plans
(5) consent.

3.1 PRESENTING COMPLAINT

In addition to determining the nature of the presenting complaint, that is, whether there is an aesthetic or functional problem, questions such as 'Why have you come to see me today?' or 'What is the problem with your teeth as far as you are concerned?' will help to determine factors that may have an influence on the complexity of any subsequent treatment plan. Such factors will include the following:

1. The degree of understanding the patient has of their own orthodontic problem.

2. How concerned they are about the problem. This may become evident either from their verbal response, or via their body language. For instance, do they attempt to suppress a smile rather than show grossly malaligned upper incisors, and yet remain reluctant to admit they are of concern? Is their verbal response suggestive perhaps of an obsession with only a minor malalignment or are they completely unaware of the condition?

3. Who instigated the referral. It has been shown that a large proportion of orthodontic referrals are instigated by the referring dentist.[1] A much smaller number are due to parent or patient demand. If the referral has been patient driven it is likely that a greater degree of motivation will be present and the patient is more likely to cooperate with any proposed treatment. However, a general dental practitioner-instigated referral may indicate a functional disturbance rather than an aesthetic problem, which may not be evident to the patient.

4. In describing their complaint, patients will often give helpful clues as to the possible aetiology of their malocclusion, the likely treatment that is required, how difficult it is going to be to treat, the probable long term stability of such treatment, and an indication as to the degree of priority that should be given to their malocclusion. For example, in describing an increased overjet they may indicate that they have a recessive chin and that a relative of their was treated with a 'jaw operation'. This may point the clinician in the direction of a possible skeletal factor in the

aetiology of the malocclusion. Priority may be given to the treatment of such an individual if they were at the start of their pubertal growth spurt and if it was felt that the use of a functional appliance would treat the malocclusion successfully, obviating the need for later surgery. Conversely, the complaint of a recently drifting upper central incisor in an adult, whilst indicating periodontal disease as the most likely aetiological agent, would mean delaying orthodontic treatment until the periodontal condition had been treated. Subsequent orthodontic correction will usually be straightforward, but retention at the end of active treatment will be needed indefinitely, either on a part- or full time basis.

5. The taking of a history will never in itself diagnose a case and determine the treatment objectives and possible treatment plans. However, it will greatly assist in the formulation of such objectives and plans to suit the needs of the individual patient.

3.2 PAST MEDICAL HISTORY

The following list is a typical example of a medical history which might be asked.

1. Have you any history of heart problems?
2. Have you any history of chest problems?
3. Have you ever had jaundice or hepatitis?
4. Are you taking any tablets, pills, or other medicines prescribed by your doctor?
5. Are you allergic to anything such as penicillin?
6. Do you bleed excessively if you cut yourself?
7. Have you ever been into hospital for any reason?
8. Do you have any experience of local or general anaesthesia?
9. Do you suffer from any other illnesses, such as diabetes or epilepsy, not already covered?
10. If radiographs are to be obtained later in the examination, female patients of childbearing age should be asked if they are likely to be pregnant.

Essentially, asking the above history is aimed at determining the following.

1. Are there any contraindications to appliance wear? For example, a poorly controlled *grand mal* epileptic may best be treated by fixed appliances rather than removable appliances. Headgear wear might also be contraindicated. A patient with a heart murmur who is to be treated with fixed appliances may best be treated using only bonded attachments and not bands, and will require antibiotic prophylaxis prior to extractions. The use of prophylactic antibiotics for fixed appliance placement in such cases is still controversial. Even when oral hygiene standards are excellent the placement of orthodontic bands has been shown to produce a bacteraemia in approximately 10 per cent of patients.[2] However, the extent of the bacteraemia necessary to lead to bacterial endocarditis is unknown. In addition, the use of antibiotics is not entirely risk free. If there is any doubt over the patient's suitability for fixed appliances and the need for antibiotic cover, contact should be made with the patient's general physician or cardiologist for advice, and certainly only bonded attachments used.

2. Are preoperative precautions necessary for any minor oral surgical procedures required as part of the orthodontic treatment? This might include antibiotic cover for extractions in a patient with a heart murmur, or perhaps preoperative steroids prior to exposing a palatal canine.

3. Could a less complex treatment approach be considered for any reason such as problems with local or general anaesthetics in the past, or a bleeding disorder?

4. Are precautions needed to protect the operator and nurse during treatment? An example of a high risk patient would be one with a history of infection from such agents as hepatitis B to F, or the human immunodeficiency virus.

3.3 PAST DENTAL HISTORY

Past dental history may be a good guide to motivation. A patient who has attended the dentist regularly and has acted well on previous advice (e.g. on oral hygiene and diet) is also likely to do the same during orthodontic treatment. Patients who attend their general dental practitioner on a regular basis but have a continued high caries rate may either flagrantly ignore dietary advice or be highly susceptible to carious attack. In the former case, if dietary advice is ignored, then so might any other instructions given during orthodontic treatment. This might then have consequences for treatment progress, oral health, or both. Patients who only attend their general dentist on a casual basis also often fail to comply well with orthodontic treatment.

Those patients who are particularly anxious about dental treatment as a whole may tolerate a short course of upper removable appliance therapy, for example to procline an upper incisor over the bite. Indeed this may be part of a systematic approach, along with other simple procedures such as polishing the teeth with a rubber cup, which can be used to help the patient overcome their fears of dentistry. Anything other than very simple appliance therapy, however, should be delayed until their anxiety has been allayed using other techniques.

A previous history of orthodontic treatment is also a good guide to likely future cooperation and success. Not infrequently, patients return as adults to complete treatment they failed to cooperate with in their teenage years. If treatment is still possible, these patients often turn out to be well motivated and thus respond well to treatment. However, the implications of treatment such as headgear wear or prolonged retention post-treatment, have to be re-explored with the patient. The latter will be particularly important in adults who have returned following relapse of perhaps lower incisor alignment or overjet reduction, where orthodontic treatment was previously successfully completed. However, if relapse has occurred once it will invariably happen again and a stable orthodontic result is difficult to achieve. Such cases will require permanent retention at the end of active orthodontic treatment.

A history of specific dental problems the patient may have suffered is also helpful. For example, the history may indicate teeth of possible poor prognosis, such as those that have suffered trauma and which may be at risk of pulpal death if moved orthodontically. Such evidence of previous trauma may not be immediately apparent on intra-oral examination.

3.4 EXPLANATION OF POSSIBLE ORTHODONTIC TREATMENT PLANS

Following the taking of a formal history, along with clinical examination (see Chapters 4 and 5) and any special investigations (see Chapter 8), it will usually be possible to formulate a number of possible treatment plans for the patient and their presenting malocclusion. These can be described to the patient and parent either in increasing order of complexity, from perhaps acceptance of the malocclusion through to fixed appliance treatment in combination with surgery, or in order of appropriateness to meet the needs of the particular patient. The degree of appropriateness might be determined by factors such as motivation, ease of travelling for treatment, medical history, or severity of the malocclusion, to name but a few.

When describing treatment it is important to cover all aspects of appliance wear and not to provide different appliances once treatment is under way. Examples would include deciding to use headgear midway through the treatment, or informing the patient on completion that indefinite retention is going to be required using a bonded retainer. This will not only affect cooperation but is an essential component of informed consent. The patient and parents should be made aware of the length of treatment and the need for regular attendance, not just to see the orthodontist, but also for routine checks at their general dentist for caries and periodontal disease.

Once all this has been explained and both the patient and parent have had the opportunity to ask any questions they might have, it is worth asking them to go away and to think the various options over. They should then make contact with a decision as to their preferred treatment option, in writing. For the more complex multidisciplinary treatment plans involving either restorative dentistry or oral and maxillofacial surgery, the patient needs to be reviewed with a specialist from the appropriate discipline, in order to confirm or modify the various treatment options available.

3.5 CONSENT

Without obtaining consent prior to the examination or treatment of any patient, a practitioner could be deemed liable for 'assault to the person'.[3] The patient's informed consent must be obtained before any procedure other than an examination is undertaken. Essentially there are three types of consent:

- implied consent
- verbal consent
- written consent.

When a patient arranges an appointment for an examination, consent for this procedure is implied. Similarly for children, consent is implied if the appointment for the child has been made by the parent or legal guardian. However, before proceeding to any special investigation as part of this examination (e.g. the taking of radiographs or photographs), the patient or parent must be informed of the necessity for the proposed procedure. With radiographs it is usually sufficient to state that they are about to be taken, or that the patient is being sent for a radiograph to be taken. In the case of patients under the age of 16 years the parent should be informed before proceeding.

Prior to embarking upon treatment of any kind it is necessary for the practitioner to explain to the patient or parent what the treatment will entail, including where possible the likely benefits and risks involved (risk/benefit analysis). It would be inappropriate and probably impossible to explain all of the benefits and possible side-effects to a patient or parent and a common-sense approach is usually required. Too much information might begin to confuse the patient. Too little and not only might cooperation with treatment be compromised, but there would be a lack of informed consent for treatment to commence. It is important to explain the various aspects of the treatment to the patient in a language and using terminology which they can understand. The aims of the treatment should be explained along with a realistic treatment outcome and the necessary effort which has to be made by the patient if this is to be achieved. This will include maintaining a good standard of plaque control, regular attendance for appliance adjustment, and wearing intra-oral elastics or headgear as is necessary. When consent is either implied or verbal, it is best done in the presence of a third party such as the dental nurse. For particularly complex procedures, or those which might involve large sums of money being paid by the patient, written consent should be obtained. In such cases not only must the details of the treatment such as extractions, use of headgear, and the need for retainers be described, but in the case of fees being paid the total sum, including when and how it is be paid, also needs to be agreed.

If a patient should get part way through a course of orthodontic treatment and request discontinuation of treatment, then the possible side-effects should once again be explained to the patient or parent. The fact that treatment is now being declined should be entered in the patients records and be countersigned by the patient or parent in the case of children under 16 years of age.[4]

Summary of the patient and parent interview

The aim of the interview is to determine the concerns of the patient and to elucidate any factors that may have an influence on the type of orthodontic treatment that could be offered. In addition, the requirements of treatment can be explained to the patient. The important points to consider are

(1) the presenting complaint;
(2) past medical history;
(3) past dental history;
(4) explanation of the possible treatment options;
(5) consent.

Objectives

1. Record all aspects of the patient's medical and dental history
2. Identify which features are of concern to the patient/parents
3. Confirm the consent
4. Confirm the risks/benefits with the parent/patient

REFERENCES

1. Shaw, W. C., Gabe, M. J., and Jones, B. M. (1979). The expectations of orthodontic patients in South Wales and St Louis, Missouri. *British Journal of Orthodontics*, **6**, 203–5.
2. McLaughlin, J. O., Coulter W. A., Coffey A., and Burden, D. J. (1996). The incidence of bacteremia after orthodontic banding. *American Journal of Orthodontics and Dentofacial Orthopedics*, **109**, 639–44.
3. Seear, J. (1981). *Law and ethics in dentistry*. Wright-PSG, Bristol.
4. Rowe, A. H. R. (1994). Consent. *Dental Update*, **21**, 188–90.

4

Extra-oral examination

Clinical examination should begin as the patient enters the surgery. They will be completely unaware that the examination will have begun and this provides an opportune moment to view the extra-oral features at rest and in function. Specifically, the following features can be assessed, preferably in the order listed:

(1) dental base relationship
  - (a) anteroposterior
  - (b) vertical
  - (c) lateral/transverse
(2) soft tissues
  - (a) lip morphology
  - (b) lip competence
  - (c) anterior oral seal
  - (d) resting lip length and upper incisor coverage
  - (e) the functional behaviour of the tongue.

Once seated and following the patient and parent interview the full extra-oral examination can commence.

4.1 DENTAL BASE RELATIONSHIP

The dental bases comprise the maxilla and mandible and are the bones that support the teeth and alveolar processes. There is no distinct anatomical boundary between the dental base and alveolar process but functionally the alveolar process can be regarded as comprising the bone whose development and existence depends on the presence of the teeth and whose form is influenced by the position of the teeth. When teeth are moved the alveolar process will undergo remodelling to accommodate this movement, a process which is known as dento-alveolar adaptation. The size and position of the underlying dental bases at this stage will remain unaffected. Similarly if teeth are extracted, the now redundant alveolar bone will undergo resorption, while the basal bone will remain unaltered.

Dental arch form and size are influenced by dental base form and size, although the orofacial musculature also plays an important part in moulding the form of the arches (see Chapter 2). If, for example, the mandible is recessive relative to the maxilla, the upper and lower incisors may be in a relatively normal relationship with each other under the action of the surrounding soft tissues. The lower incisors may be proclined due to the action of the lips and tongue and thereby still remain in contact with the upper incisors. This is known as dento-alveolar compensation, and may greatly simplify orthodontic treatment. In some cases, where dento-alveolar compensation for an underlying skeletal discrepancy has not occurred, the malocclusion may be deemed as being beyond treatment with orthodontic appliances alone, requiring instead a combined surgical and orthodontic treatment approach. In other instances there may be the potential for orthodontic treatment to correct the malocclusion by inducing such dento-alveolar compensation. Dento-alveolar compensation occurs in all three planes of space: anteroposterior, vertical, and transverse.

The effect of this close relationship between skeletal and soft tissue patterns, in the aetiology and subsequent diagnosis of a malocclusion, serves to illustrate how many of the factors involved in the malocclusion are interlinked. No single diagnostic feature can be used to determine aetiology and hence any necessary treatment plan. The purpose of the extra-oral examination is to assess both the skeletal and soft tissue relationships with a view to determining their individual and combined effects on the occlusion.

4.1.1 Clinical examination

Skeletal relationship

Dental base relationships are assessed in three planes of space: sagittal, vertical, and transverse.

Sagittal skeletal relationship

In order to carry out the extra-oral examination the patient should sit unsupported in the chair with the head in the free-postural position (Fig. 4.1). In this way the Frankfort plane, a line joining the upper border of the external auditory meatus and the lower border of the soft tissue orbit, should be approximately horizontal, that is, parallel with the floor. It is also important to make the assessment of skeletal relationship with the teeth in centric occlusion. In cases where there is an anteroposterior displacement when the patient closes into a position of maximum intercuspation (see Chapter 6), it is also worth assessing skeletal pattern with the patient in the pre-displaced position.

The clinical assessment is made using the index and middle finger of one hand as shown in Fig. 4.2. The aim is to palpate the anterior borders of both the maxilla and mandible and so determine their relationship, one to the other. The tip of the index finger

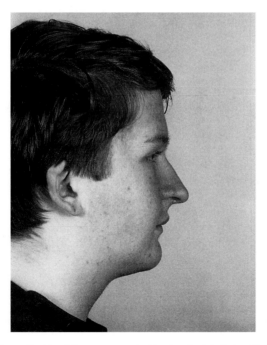

Fig. 4.1 The patient is sitting unsupported in the dental chair with the head in the free-postural position.

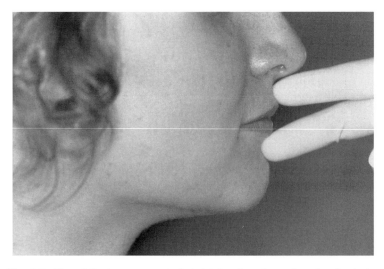

Fig. 4.2 The clinical assessment of skeletal pattern is made using the index and middle finger of one hand. In this case a class I skeletal pattern is assessed as being present when the middle finger is 2–3 mm closer to the patient than the index finger.

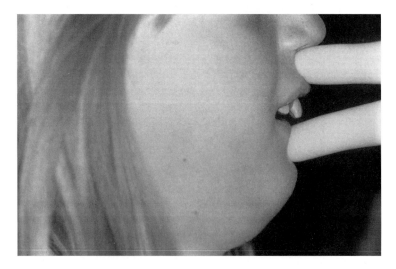

Fig. 4.3 A class II skeletal pattern is assessed as being present when the middle finger is 4 mm or more closer to the patient than the index finger.

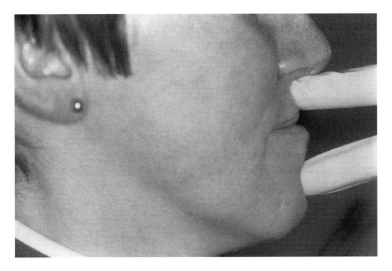

Fig. 4.4 A class III skeletal pattern is assessed as being present when the middle finger is less than 2–3 mm closer to the patient than the index finger.

is placed in the concavity between the base of the nose and the vermilion border of the upper lip, while the tip of the middle finger is placed in the concavity between the vermilion border of the lower lip and the bony chin. Retraction of the lips has been advocated in order to more fully palpate the bony structures and thereby provide a more accurate determination of the position of the mandible and maxilla. However, in most instances this does nothing but obscure the finger tips, making the assessment of the anteroposterior skeletal relationships even more difficult.

The anteroposterior relation of the dental bases is grouped into three classes, I, II, and III.

- Class I skeletal pattern – the tip of the middle finger (on the anterior border of the mandible) will be 2–3 mm closer to the patient than the tip of the index finger (on the maxilla) (Fig. 4.2). This is the normal anteroposterior relationship between the maxilla and the mandible.

- Class II skeletal pattern – the tip of the middle finger (on the anterior border of the mandible) will be 4 mm or more closer to the patient than the tip of the index finger (on the maxilla) (Fig. 4.3). The mandible is posteriorly placed in relation to the maxilla.

- Class III skeletal pattern – the tip of the index finger (on the anterior border maxilla) will be 2–3 mm closer toward the patient than the tip of the middle finger (on the anterior border of the mandible) (Fig. 4.4). The maxilla is posteriorly placed in relation to the mandible.

The description of class II and class III skeletal relationships is often supplemented by the terms mild, moderate, or severe. These are somewhat arbitrary terms varying from clinician to clinician. Generally, if the anteroposterior discrepancy is mild, the prognosis for orthodontic correction of the associated malocclusion is good. A severe discrepancy may not be amenable to orthodontic treatment as the basal bone discrepancy is likely to be the principal agent in the aetiology of the malocclusion. Such cases will often require a combined orthodontic and surgical approach to treatment. A class II division 1 incisor relationship on a mild class II skeletal base may readily be treated to become a class I incisor relationship, perhaps with removable or fixed appliances. In this case tipping the upper incisors palatally to meet the lower incisors to create a class I incisor relationship will produce a good result. The same incisor relationship on a moderate class II skeletal base may be treatable with fixed appliances allowing bodily retraction of the incisors, whereas if removable appliances were to be used it would lead to retroclination of the upper incisors to create a class II division 2 incisor relationship (Fig. 4.5). On a severe class II skeletal base even fixed appliances would be inappropriate and a combined orthodontic and surgical approach may be required. The orthodontic treatment will deal with the alignment of the teeth within their respective arches, while the surgery will correct the severe class II skeletal discrepancy.

Vertical relationships
With the patient sitting in the chair in the same position as described previously, the vertical skeletal relationship is assessed in two ways, angularly and linearly

Angular relationship An angular assessment is made between the two skeletal bases when observing the patient in profile. The accepted reference plane for the mandible is its lower border, whilst for the maxilla it is a line passing through both the anterior and

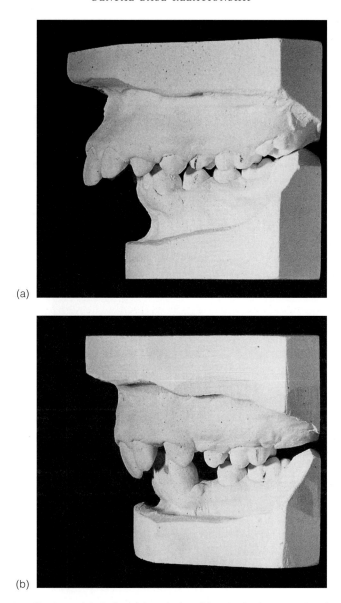

(a)

(b)

Fig. 4.5 Study models before (a) and after (b) orthodontic treatment, demonstrating how inappropriate treatment of a class II division 1 incisor relationship on a moderate class II skeletal base with a removable appliance has created a class II division 2 incisor relationship.

posterior nasal spines (Fig. 4.6). At the chairside it is impossible to
see this maxillary plane, as not only is it a midline structure, but
the maxilla is obscured by the overlying soft tissues. The maxillary
plane can only be visualized accurately on a lateral skull radiograph. No such problem exists with the mandible as its lower
border forms the mandibular plane and is visualized by holding the
index finger in contact with it, as illustrated in Fig. 4.7. The chair-
side substitute for the maxillary plane is the Frankfort plane, visualized by imagining a line between two points, namely the upper
border of the external auditory meatus and the lower border of the
orbit. In the clinic it is therefore possible to determine the angle
made between the Frankfort plane and the mandibular plane. The
normal Frankfort–mandibular planes angle is $27 \pm 5°$ and with a
little experience it is easy to estimate whether the angle is average,

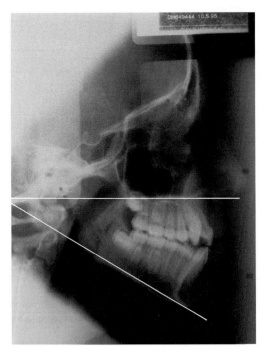

Fig. 4.6 A lateral skull radiograph showing the mandibular and maxillary
planes. The latter cannot be assessed clinically and the Frankfort plane is therefore used in the absence of a radiograph.

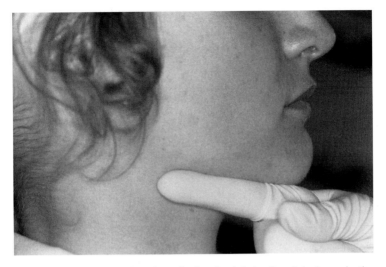

Fig. 4.7   The mandibular plane is easily visualized during the clinical examination.

increased, or decreased. A protractor can be used, but a simpler estimate is to consider the point of intersection of the two lines. Normally this should be in the region of the occiput on the patient's head. If the angle is increased, the visualized intersect will be anterior to this, and *vice versa* if the angle is decreased (Fig. 4.8). Assessment of the angle between the mandible and maxilla, as with other aspects of the clinical examination, will help

(1) the determination of the possible aetiology of the malocclusion;
(2) to predict the likely direction of continued mandibular growth (see Chapter 2);
(3) the clinician to build up a mental picture of the malocclusion;
(4) to determine possible treatment plans.

For example, a case described as having a high angle, that is, where the angle between the mandible and maxilla is increased (Fig. 4.9), may be associated with a reduced overbite or even an anterior open bite (see later in Chapter 5). The appearance on the radiograph may suggest a possible backwards growth rotation of the mandible, which may further reduce the overbite with time. Such information will help the clinician to build up a mental picture, not only of what the case is like at present, but also how it

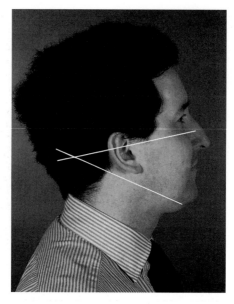

Fig. 4.8 This patient can be seen with a high Frankfort mandibular planes angle. Notice how the two planes intersect on the region of the skull in front of the occiput.

may alter in the future with continued facial growth, and how treatment planning should proceed once the remainder of the clinical examination has been completed.

Linear relationship   The aim of the linear assessment of vertical skeletal relationship is to determine the anterior lower face height in relation to total face height.

The patient is usually examined either in profile, or full face from directly in front. Total face height is assessed as the distance between the lower border of the bony chin and a point midway between the eyebrows, known as Glabella. The anterior lower face height is the distance between the lower border of the bony chin and the base of the columella, that is, where the nose meets the upper lip in the midline. Although these distances can be measured using a millimetre rule, it is more usual to determine the percentage the anterior lower face height forms of the total anterior face height. Normally it will account for 50 per cent of the total

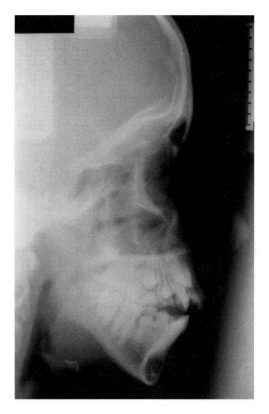

Fig. 4.9 Lateral skull radiograph illustrating an increased maxillary–mandibular planes angle (MMA) (see also growth rotations in Chapter 8).

(Fig. 4.10). Both angular and linear dimensions of the facial skeleton are assessed because there is not necessarily a direct correlation between the two. For instance it is not unusual for the anterior lower face height to be increased and yet the Frankfort–mandibular planes angle to be reduced, and *vice versa*. The Frankfort–mandibular planes angle is not a measure of anterior lower face height but a ratio between posterior lower face height and anterior lower face height (Fig. 4.11).

Transverse relationship
Transverse skeletal discrepancies are often difficult to assess, especially if the discrepancy is bilateral and therefore symmetrical. They

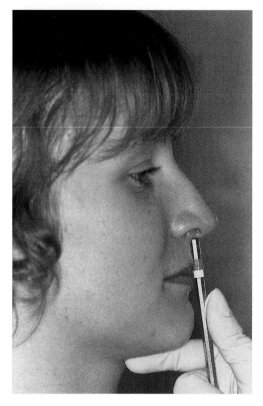

Fig. 4.10 The anterior lower face height is assessed as the distance between the base of the bony chin (Menton) and the base of the columella of the nose. Anterior lower face height normally comprises 50–55 per cent of the total anterior face height. Total anterior face height is the distance between the base of the bony chin (Menton) and a point between the eyebrows known as Glabella.

are best viewed either by looking at the patient from above and behind, or by viewing the face from directly in front. It should be noted that we all have some degree of facial asymmetry and as such, a mild discrepancy can be regarded as perfectly normal.

Transverse skeletal malrelationships may be due to:

(1) a difference in transverse size between two symmetrical skeletal bases (i.e. mandible and maxilla);

(2) a true asymmetry in one or both of the skeletal bases; or

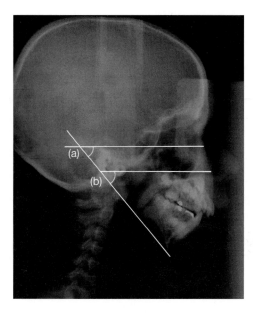

Fig. 4.11 Lateral skull radiograph illustrating how the angles (a) FMPA and MMA (b) are a measure of the ratio between anterior and posterior lower face height and not a direct measure of anterior lower face height. In this case, with rheumatoid arthritis of the temporomandibular joints, there is a marked ante-gonal notch.

(3) an incorrect anteroposterior relationship of the skeletal bases rather than a difference in size between the upper and lower jaws. For example, if the articulation of the mandible with the cranial base is more anterior than normal this can lead to a class III anteroposterior skeletal relationship. In addition a more posterior and thus wider part of the mandible will be opposing an anterior and hence narrower part of the maxilla. It is for this reason that class III skeletal relationships are often associated with bilateral posterior crossbites.

The effect on the occlusion of a mild skeletal asymmetry is in most instances negated by the action of the soft tissues. Moulding of the dento-alveolar complex will often result in correct transverse interocclusal relationships of the teeth, even in the presence of a mild asymmetry. However, a more marked transverse skeletal discrepancy may result in the development of a posterior crossbite. The development of a unilateral posterior crossbite as a result of a

digit sucking habit has been discussed previously (Chapter 2).
Such a crossbite is usually associated with a displacement on
closing into centric occlusion. In the case of skeletal asymmetries a
unilateral crossbite, where present, is not usually associated with
such a displacement. If the transverse discrepancy between the
maxilla and the mandible is symmetrical then a unilateral crossbite with a displacement may be present, but as mentioned previously, there may not be a crossbite at all if there has been
sufficient dento-alveolar compensation. When the transverse discrepancy between the arches is more marked and symmetrical, the
effect on the occlusion is usually to create a bilateral posterior
crossbite, but once again without a displacement. The presence or
absence of a displacement associated with any crossbite is most
important, since not only does it assist in the determination of the
need for orthodontic treatment, but also in the likely prognosis for
correction of the crossbite. This will be discussed further in
Chapter 5 (Intra-oral examination).

4.2 SOFT TISSUES

Examination of the soft tissues both in form and function can be
fraught with difficulties, especially in the child patient, and so
should once again begin as the patient enters the surgery. At this
time the patient is likely to be unaware that the examination is in
progress and the true position of the lips and tongue relative to the
teeth can be noted, both at rest and in function. Once the formal
clinical examination begins, soft tissue assessment can be difficult
in some patients. The features to be noted in both the casual and
formal examination are:

(1) lip morphology

(2) lip competence

(3) anterior oral seal

(4) resting lip length and upper incisor coverage

(5) the tongue.

Although an intra-oral feature, the tongue will be described under
extra-oral features, for convenience.

4.2.1 Clinical examination

When formally examining the soft tissues the patient can be examined with the head in an unsupported free-postural position, as for the examination of skeletal pattern. Alternatively the patient may be permitted to rest their head against the headrest of the chair. What is important is that the patient is sitting upright and the head is not tipped back. This can lead to the normal position of the lips being misdiagnosed, both with respect to the incisors and lip competence. Generally, the patient should be asked to relax in order to assess lip form and also their resting position. In some patients, particularly those with a very active lower lip muscle, this can be extremely difficult to achieve. However, gentle, yet definite contact with the skin overlying this area with the clinicians fingers often appears to reduce this contraction.

Once relaxed and when no apparent signs of muscle activity are visible, the lips may be judged to be competent or incompetent. If they are competent the presence of circum-oral muscle contraction should be looked for, to determine whether they in fact have incompetent lips which are habitually held together. The resting position of the lower lip in relation to the upper incisors should be noted. If the lips are competent then the clinician should gently lift the upper lip in order to be able to see where the lower lip rests relative to the crowns of the four upper incisors.

Once the soft tissues have been assessed at rest, they should then be assessed in function. In order to do this the patient should be instructed to lick their lips and swallow. If the patient is particularly anxious at this time a glass of water will make this part of the examination easier. During swallowing the method by which the patient achieves an anterior oral seal should be determined. Whilst repeating the procedure the lower lip can be gently pulled forwards in order to observe the behaviour of the tongue during swallowing.

The major problem with any examination of the soft tissues is that examination itself may modify soft tissue behaviour. Whereas soft tissue examination is usually straightforward, for some patients the soft tissues seem almost to have a mind of their own as soon as the clinician begins to look at them!

The significance of the soft tissues has been discussed in Chapter 2 in the aetiology of malocclusion. The specific details of the soft tissues will now be assessed.

Lip morphology

Whereas hard tissues can easily be quantified, both in terms of size and position, such an assessment of the soft tissues is difficult to make. The teeth are known to assume a position of balance between the forces applied to them from the lips and cheeks on one side, and the tongue on the other. The forces are those applied at rest as well as during function. Lip morphology will therefore affect tooth position. Lips that are full and everted are usually associated with proclined upper and lower labial segment teeth or bimaxillary proclination (Fig. 4.12). Lips that are relatively thin and yet active may instead be associated with retroclined upper and lower incisors or bimaxillary retroclination. In both instances it must be remembered that the teeth have adopted a position of balance and any attempt to move them, either labially or lingually, is likely to be prone to relapse. That is not to say that their alignment or the interincisal angle cannot be altered and the correction remain stable.

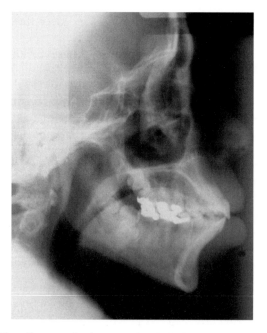

Fig. 4.12   Bimaxillary proclination associated with full and everted lips.

Lip competence

Although it has been suggested that the position of the upper and lower incisors is dictated by the morphology of the lips, this factor alone is not responsible for their position. In the child patient it is common for the lips to be apart at rest, and sometimes during function. Such lips are described as incompetent. As a child progresses through to the teenage years, increasing soft tissue maturity usually means the lips become competent with age. For the older child, and certainly for adult patients, it is socially more acceptable for the lips to be held together at rest. If such a patient has incompetent lips they may demonstrate increased contraction of the circum-oral musculature in order to habitually keep the lips together. Clinically this is usually witnessed as puckering of the skin over the chin point due to increased activity in the mentalis muscle. Such cases are described as having incompetent lips which are habitually held together. Lip incompetence can be due to:

(1) short resting lip length;

(2) an increased anterior lower face height such that the lips are unable to contact each other;

(3) a large anteroposterior skeletal discrepancy, usually class II; or

(4) interposition of the teeth between the lips in the absence of a skeletal discrepancy. This is most commonly seen in class II division 1 incisor relationships where the upper incisors are protruding between the upper and the lower lip.

The significance of recording lip competence/incompetence is to highlight the possible causes. A short resting lip length, an increased anterior lower face height, and a severe anteroposterior skeletal discrepancy cannot be altered by orthodontic means. Where the incisor teeth interpose between the upper and lower lips, orthodontic treatment to correct their position may enable the lips to become competent. Orthodontic treatment can also be used to correct a mild anteroposterior skeletal discrepancy related to lip incompetence. If the skeletal discrepancy, either sagittal or vertical, is severe then lip competence may only be achieved following orthognathic surgery. Whereas lip competence is important in affecting tooth position via the resting position of the lips, incompetence may also lead the patient to adopt alternative soft tissue patterns of behaviour in order to attain an anterior oral seal during swallowing, which in turn may further influence tooth position.

Anterior oral seal

During the first or oral phase of normal swallowing the following sequence of events is said to occur:

(1) a lip seal is obtained with minimal muscular effort;
(2) the tip of the tongue is lightly applied to the palatal mucosa just behind the upper incisor teeth;
(3) the teeth are brought lightly into occlusion; and
(4) the floor of the mouth is elevated by the action of the mylohyoid muscle, bringing the remainder of the tongue into contact with the hard palate so that the bolus of food is passed into the pharynx.

Lip to lip contact creates the anterior oral seal required to prevent the contents of the mouth from being expelled during swallowing. If a patient has incompetent lips, which cannot be brought into contact by increased circum-oral muscle activity, then an anterior oral seal must be achieved by another method. The patient is described as adopting an adaptive anterior oral seal or adaptive swallowing behaviour (see Glossary). These adaptive methods include the following:

Tongue to lower lip swallow
This is commonly seen in a class II division 1 incisor relationship and a diagnostic clue as to its presence is to look closely at the overbite (see Chapter 2). Although this may be increased it is usually just incomplete. This adaptive oral seal can usually be seen in action either by casual observation of the patient during swallowing or by asking them to lick their lips and swallow. At the same time the clinician needs to gently pull the lower lip forwards. The tongue can usually be seen to be overlying the incisal edges of the lower incisors, even though the teeth may be lightly in occlusion. A tongue to lower lip swallow may also be seen in cases where there is a persistent digit sucking habit with an associated anterior open bite. In such cases there will usually be an asymmetric anterior open bite and the diagnostic feature of an increased but just incomplete overbite will not be present.

Lower lip to palate
This is once again commonly seen in class II division 1 incisor relationships but usually in association with a class II skeletal discrepancy. This mode of adaptive swallowing is usually more readily noticeable than the previous tongue to lower lip swallowing behaviour. In this instance the overbite can be increased and complete to the palate.

Tongue to upper lip
This is most often seen in patients with a class III incisor relationship and where there is a moderate to severe class III skeletal base relationship.

Mandibular posture with a lip to lip seal
In cases with a moderate Class II skeletal base the patient may be able to achieve a lip to lip anterior oral seal by posturing the mandible forwards. On casual observation and when initially meeting a patient such mandibular posturing will not be immediately obvious. Only by performing a thorough clinical examination will it become apparent that the patient has an increased overjet. This will be seen when the patient is instructed to bring the teeth into contact with the mandibular condyles in their retruded position within the glenoid fossae.

Which adaptive behaviour a patient utilizes will largely depend on their skeletal, soft tissue, and occlusal features. Generally a patient will assume the method which most easily and comfortably affords an anterior oral seal. Common to all patterns of adaptive swallowing is that correction of the malocclusion will lead to a cessation of adaptive swallowing behaviour and the attainment of a lip to lip anterior oral seal during swallowing.

Resting lip length and upper incisor coverage

The significance of the assessment of upper incisor coverage by the lips is threefold.

1. Is the resting lip position implicated in the aetiology of the malocclusion? In cases where the lips are incompetent and the upper incisors are proclined and outside lower lip control, it is necessary to determine whether the lack of coverage of the upper incisors is due to incompetent lips. Alternatively, the lip incompetence may be due

to the position of the incisors. Following retraction of the upper incisors to reduce, for example, an overjet in a class II division 1 incisor relationship, the major determinant of stability of this tooth movement is whether the lower lip covers at least the incisal third of the crowns of the upper incisors at rest. If lip incompetence is implicated in the aetiology of the incisor position, then orthodontic treatment may reduce the overjet, but the lips will remain incompetent. If at least the incisal third of the upper incisor crowns are not subsequently controlled by the lower lip at rest, then overjet reduction will relapse, since the major aetiological agent is still operating. If on the other hand the upper incisors are interposing between the lips, which are incompetent as a result, then overjet reduction in such a case is likely to remain stable. This is because post-treatment, the patient will have competent lips, and the lower lip will cover the all important incisal third of the crowns of the upper incisors.

Lower lip position is also implicated in the aetiology of class II division 2 incisor relationships, as discussed in Chapter 2. In particular the position of the lower lip line is important. In cases where all four upper incisor teeth are retroclined the lower lip is usually seen to be resting high on the crowns of these teeth if the upper lip is lifted during the clinical examination (Fig. 4.13). In the classical description of the class II division 2 incisor relationship the upper central incisors are retroclined, whilst the upper lateral incisors are proclined, mesially angulated, and mesiolabially rotated. The reason the upper central incisors are retroclined and the upper lateral incisors are proclined is because the high lower lip line controls the longer crowns of the central incisors, but is unable to control the shorter crowns of the upper lateral incisors (Fig. 4.14).

2. Will altering the incisor position enable the lower lip to cover at least the incisal third of the crown of the upper incisors? This would maintain their corrected position following orthodontic treatment. As discussed in the previous section, lower lip coverage of the upper incisors is not only implicated in the aetiology of incisor position prior to treatment but is of the utmost importance in maintaining corrected incisor positions and, in particular, in overjet reduction. The likelihood of coverage of at least a third of the crowns of the upper incisors by the lower lip needs to be assessed before commencing orthodontic treatment. If this cannot

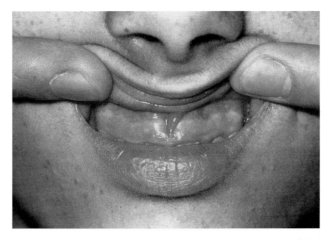

Fig. 4.13 Retraction of the upper lip in this class II division 2 incisor relationship shows how there is a high lower lip line covering most of the upper incisor crowns.

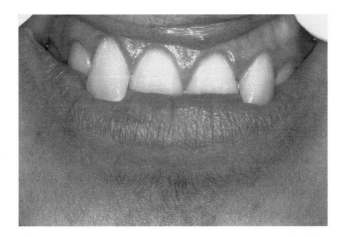

Fig. 4.14 The lower lip line in this class II division 2 incisor relationship is high relative to the upper central incisors but is not controlling the upper lateral incisors, which as a consequence are proclined, mesially angulated, and mesio-labially rotated.

be achieved, overjet reduction will not be stable and the patient must be made aware of this before proceeding with treatment.

3. Does the upper lip cover the upper incisors adequately at rest and in function? Ideally the upper lip should cover most of the upper incisor crown at rest and in function with no more than approximately 3–5 mm of upper incisor crown being visible. There are, however, variations between the sexes and with age, with more of the lower incisors being visible as the individual ages.[1] When the patient smiles the upper incisors should be exposed, but an excessive amount of the upper labial gingivae should not be visible. Excessive exposure of the gingivae at rest, or in function, such as when smiling, is unaesthetic. It is often, but not always, related to inadequate upper lip length and in addition, the patient may have what is often termed a characteristic 'roller-blind' upper lip, which appears to retract readily on smiling. If this is the case and it is the patient's principal complaint, then orthodontic treatment alone may not deal with the problem and a surgical approach to impact the maxilla may be required.

Nasolabial angle

It can be extremely useful to assess the form of the soft tissues beneath the nares, particularly in profile. Many claims are made regarding the effects of orthodontic treatment on this area. In particular, emphasis is placed on the possible deleterious effects on the nasolabial angle following orthodontic treatment involving extractions. It is often said that following such extraction treatment the upper lip is retracted relative to the nose and the nasolabial angle becomes more obtuse. Current research findings do not always support this view and it is not as yet possible to predict accurately the likely effects of treatment.

The commonly used descriptions of the nasolabial angle are 'acceptable', 'acute', or 'obtuse'.

The protrusion of the upper and lower lips in repose

A line has been identified when viewing the facial profile, which joins the tip of the nose to the soft tissue pogonion. It has been suggested that the lips should lie on or in front of this line for an attractive profile. Indeed the original data stem from investigations as to why a model's facial appearance is attractive.[2] The effect of orthodontic treatment on their position is controversial. However, as an aid to describing the soft tissues it is helpful to describe the position of the lips with respect to this line.

An additional feature to identify is muscle tone of the lips. This can vary from highly active to extremely flaccid lips, where there appears little tone. The latter is usually associated with proclination of both upper and lower labial segments. Alternatively the lips, the lower in particular, can show a great deal of muscle activity during function. In such cases a strap-like lower lip will indicate a high level of muscular activity and can produce retroclination of the lower labial segment.

4.3 TEMPOROMANDIBULAR JOINTS AND MUSCLES OF MASTICATION

The temporomandibular joint (TMJ) is considered in Chapter 6. The joints and the masticatory muscles should be examined prior to orthodontic treatment:

(1) to assess whether there is any tenderness in the joints or muscles, or any deviations of the mandible on opening or closing which could be attributed to the malocclusion; and

(2) for medico-legal reasons, to ensure no muscle or joint problems can be attributed to the orthodontics either during or after treatment (see Chapter 9).

The temporomandibular joints are best examined from above and behind the patient. It is useful to rest the first two fingers of each hand gently over the joints, to assess any tenderness and also to palpate for any crepitus in the joints on opening and closing the mandible. At the same time the chin point is observed during mandibular movements in order to determine whether there are any deviations on opening or closing. This examination is usually greatly assisted by the patient's history of the presenting problems, if any. Further abnormalities such as disc trapping can be inferred by this clinical examination and assist in the understanding of any abnormality. Identification of any abnormal movements of either hard or soft tissues during this examination of the joints may imply a functional derangement requiring further investigation.

The masticatory muscles in some instances can be observed indirectly, otherwise they can be palpated. Both temporalis and masseter can be observed in function, and in patients who indulge in parafunctional habits such as bruxism the masseters may undergo hypertrophy. This may indicate an excessive loading of the dental structures which may make orthodontic treatment difficult and may be associated with increased occlusal wear in the dentition. Further simple investigations of the major muscles can be undertaken by palpating the main muscle mass. An inflamed muscle, perhaps as a consequence of increased usage, may be very tender due to the build-up of inflammatory products such as lactic acid or potassium ions.[3]

Summary of the extra-oral examination

The four important components of the extra-oral examination are listed below.

1. Skeletal relationships
   (a) Sagittal – Classes I, II and III. The latter two are subdivided into mild, moderate, and severe
   (b) Vertical – described using angles, namely the Frankfort–mandibular planes angle (FMPA) clinically, and maxillary – mandibular planes angle (MMPA) radiographically
   (c) Transverse – described in terms of relative narrowness and symmetry or asymmetry

2. Soft tissues
   (a) Lip morphology
   (b) Lip competence
   (c) Anterior oral seal
   (d) Resting lip length and upper incisor coverage
   (e) Nasolabial angle
   (f) Protrusion of the lips in repose

3. Swallowing patterns
   (a) Lip to lip
   (b) Tongue to lower lip
   (c) Lower lip to palate
   (d) Tongue to upper lip
   (e) Mandibular posture with a lip to lip seal

4. Temporomandibular joints and muscles of mastication

Objectives

1. Recall the definitions of skeletal base including vertical, antero-posterior and lateral
2. List all the features of lip morphology
3. List the types of swallowing behaviour

REFERENCES

1. Vig, R. G. and Brundo, G. C. (1978). The kinetics of anterior tooth display. *Journal of Prosthetic Dentistry*, **39**, 502–4.
2. Williams, R. (1969). The diagnostic line. *American Journal of Orthodontics*, **55**, 458–76.
3. Fock, S. and Mense, S. (1976). Excitatory effects of 5-hydroxytryptamine, histamine and potassium ions on muscular group IV afferent units: a comparison with bradykinin. *Brain Research*, **105**, 459–69.

5

Intra-oral examination

The purpose of the intra-oral examination is:

(1) to assess the patient's presenting complaint;
(2) to help identify the aetiology of the malocclusion;
(3) to determine how other factors such as caries and periodontal disease might modify any subsequent treatment plan; and
(4) to identify potential treatment plans which might be used to treat the malocclusion.

Whenever an orthodontic examination is performed it should be completed in a logical and systematic fashion so that no aspect of the examination is omitted. By using such a sequence, a mental picture of the malocclusion can be formulated which, with experience, will help in the formulation of appropriate treatment aims and thus treatment plans. A pro forma for both extra- and intra-oral examination is included in Appendix 1. The intra-oral examination will now be discussed in more detail.

5.1 TEETH AND SUPPORTING STRUCTURES

The intra-oral examination should commence with the teeth and their supporting structures. In general, any investigation of the teeth and jaws aims to determine the three Ps:

- Presence
- Position
- Pathology (e.g. caries, periodontal disease, cysts, tumours)

In addition, in orthodontics, other features specifically related to the teeth need to be ascertained, namely

- shape of the teeth
- size of the teeth
- developmental stage (i.e. whether the developmental stage of the dentition is related normally to the patient's age and perhaps, more importantly, whether the developmental stage is the same in all parts of the mouth).

At the beginning of the intra-oral examination it is essential to count the teeth as it is easy to overlook developmental absence. In the mixed dentition, mobility of deciduous teeth should be tested using a mirror handle on one side of the tooth and a finger tip on the other side (Fig. 5.1). In this way symmetry in the components of the occlusion can be determined, that is, are the teeth on opposite sides of the same arch becoming mobile at the same time and are teeth erupting at the same time? Delayed eruption on one side of the arch might indicate the developmental absence of a permanent tooth or an ectopic path of eruption.

The position of unerupted teeth should be determined by palpation, especially if as mentioned, there is a lack of symmetry in the timing of deciduous tooth loss and permanent tooth eruption within an arch. In the case of delayed eruption of an upper permanent incisor for example, the clinician should palpate both palatally

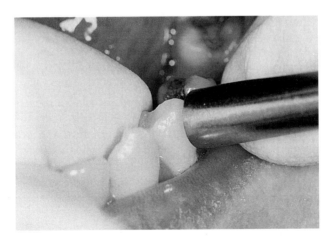

Fig. 5.1 Testing for mobility should be performed with a finger and a mirror handle opposite sides of the tooth applying controlled pressure and the resistance to movement assessed.

and labially. If there has been a history of trauma then an upper incisor might be dilacerated. In such a case it may be possible to palpate the incisor high in the labial sulcus. Although it might be possible to identify the incisal edge it may not be possible to palpate any more of the labial surface of the crown, which would indicate that the incisor is lying horizontally, or is dilacerated labially, with the crown lying in a horizontal position. Not infrequently, the upper permanent canine assumes an ectopic path of eruption and so it is necessary to palpate for this tooth, buccally, above its deciduous predecessor at approximately 9 years of age and beyond. The position of adjacent teeth may give a clue as to the position of an unerupted tooth. For instance, a feature of normal development is a distally angulated maxillary lateral incisor and spacing in the upper labial segment, prior to eruption of the upper canine.

The presence of submerging as well as retained deciduous teeth should also be noted. Submergence may be a transient stage of development with the tooth later reemerging and being naturally shed, or it may indicate the developmental absence of a permanent successor.

The presence, position, pathology, and developmental stages can be further assessed by the use of the appropriate special investigations, namely radiographs. Radiographic examination will be discussed in greater detail in Chapter 8.

The condition of all the teeth should be determined visually using a mirror, compressed air to dry the enamel surface, and where necessary, a dental probe. Bitewing radiographs may also be required. If the clinician is uncertain about the prognosis of any tooth, for example if there is caries in a first permanent molar, and the clinician is not responsible for the routine care of the patient, it may be necessary to contact the referring dentist and ask for the tooth to be investigated. Written confirmation of the prognosis (i.e. the long term prospects for the tooth) will then help in the determination of any subsequent extraction pattern.

The colour, size, and shape of the teeth should be noted. A darkened tooth, or one which appears white but opaque, may give an indication of previous trauma, as might the presence of infraction lines within the enamel when the crown is transilluminated. Special investigations in such circumstances would include pulp testing using chloroethane (ethyl chloride) on cotton wool or an electric pulp tester. A periapical radiograph will help determine whether there is any associated root pathology (e.g. root fracture) or peri-apical radiolucency perhaps due to infection or a periapical cyst.

Signs of attrition, abrasion, or erosion should be identified. Attrition may be evident on the incisal edge of an upper incisor when in crossbite and associated with a displacement on closing into centric occlusion. The presence of such attrition and a displacement (see Glossary) would be a functional indication for considering ortho-dontic treatment. Abrasion either from a tooth brush or the diet may be a finding in an adult presenting for orthodontic treatment. Of perhaps more concern is erosion, particularly in a young mouth. This can be associated with excessive consumption of fizzy drinks or possible medical disorders. If erosion is detected, its site may give a clue as to possible aetiology. Palatal erosion of most of the maxillary teeth, particularly the upper incisors, usually indicates reflux of gastric acid into the mouth. This may be due to anorexia or bulimia nervosa or gastro-oesophageal reflux disease.[1,2] Erosion of the labial as well as the palatal surfaces of the upper incisor teeth is usually due to frequent and excessive consumption of acidic food such as citrus fruit, fruit juice, or fizzy drinks.[3] Erosion due to dietary factors will necessitate dietary counselling prior to commencing orthodontic treatment. Erosion due to non-dietary factors will require investiga-tion by the patient's general medical practitioner.

Examination of the supporting tissues once again begins with a visual examination of the gingivae. Gingivitis will usually be obvious and often associated with readily visible areas of plaque accumulation. Indeed the presence or absence of gingivitis is a better guide to the normal standard of oral hygiene practised by the patient than the presence or absence of plaque, especially since patients often make an extra effort to clean their teeth before coming to the examination. If an extra effort has been made prior to the examination in a patient whose standard of oral hygiene is usually poor, then in addition to gingival inflammation, areas of enamel decalcification may be seen at the cervical margins of the teeth. Fortunately a large proportion of orthodontic patients are children in whom advanced periodontal disease is not present and the establishment of good oral hygiene measures will be sufficient to treat the gingivitis.

Occasionally, advanced bone loss in children is present due to juve-nile periodontitis. In such cases, and in adults with a history of periodontal disease, a more detailed examination will be required.

Only when existing disease has been controlled should orthodontic treatment be considered. Orthodontic treatment in the presence of progressive periodontal disease can lead to the development of acute inflammatory episodes as well as accelerate the rate of alveolar bone loss in the affected areas.[4] Teeth which have undergone marked bone loss may be incorporated into any subsequent extraction regimen as part of the orthodontic treatment. However, if such a tooth is retained and orthodontically realigned, it will require permanent retention if it is to remain in its new position at the end of treatment.

The presence of frenal attachments and their influence on the position of the teeth and gingivae should be noted. The low attachment of a fleshy upper labial frenum is often associated with a median diastema (Fig. 5.2) and may require removal either before embarking on orthodontic treatment or at the end of active treatment. The advantage of excision prior to starting orthodontic treatment is the ease of surgical access. A stated advantage of excision after completion of active tooth movement is that any scar tissue formed might help maintain closure of the diastema. Only when the frenum is particularly fleshy will it require excision. Further indications for excision might include

(1) a fraenum which is unsightly, being visible as a pendulous piece of tissue in the midline of the upper lip;

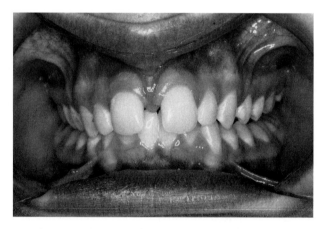

Fig. 5.2 A lower attachment of the upper labial frenum associated with a median diastema.

(2) when its presence precludes maintenance of good oral hygiene;

(3) where there is a direct attachment of the frenum at the gingival margin which might increase the rate of periodontal destruction in the presence of pre-existing periodontal disease.

5.2 LABIAL SEGMENTS

The term labial segment refers either to the four incisors or to the four incisors and both canine teeth within the arch. The order of the examination of this segment is as follows:

1. Incisor inclination – that is, **average** inclination, **proclined** or **retroclined**.
2. Crowding or spacing – that is, spaced, aligned, crowded – **mild**, **moderate** or **severe**.
3. Angulations – mesiodistal tip of the teeth.
4. Rotations.
5. Marked tooth malpositions.

Examination usually begins in the lower arch with an assessment of lower incisor inclination. This is best accomplished by asking the patient to open their mouth, and while viewing them in profile, retracting the lower lip with the thumb and holding the index finger of the same hand against the lower border of the mandible (Fig. 5.3). In this way it is possible to determine the incisor inclination with respect to the mandibular plane (lower border of the mandible). Normally the angle of the lower incisors to this plane is approximately 90°. If, during the extra-oral examination, an anteroposterior skeletal discrepancy was noted, it will be important to assess the lower incisor inclination and thereby determine the degree of dento-alveolar compensation that has taken place. Such compensation will be influenced by the soft tissues and a class I incisor relationship may be produced even in the presence of a skeletal malrelationship. Upper labial segment inclination is easily assessed by retracting the upper lip and visualizing the angle the upper incisors make with the Frankfort plane (the line joining the lower border of the orbit with the upper border of the external auditory meatus). This angle is usually 105° (±5°). A greater angle

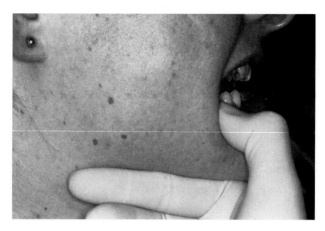

Fig. 5.3 Clinical assessment of the lower incisor inclination to the mandibular plane. The index finger is used to palpate the lower border of the mandible while the thumb is used to retract the lower lip.

would indicate proclination, and a lesser angle, retroclination of the upper incisors. The significance of the inclination of the upper labial segment becomes apparent when assessed in combination with the skeletal pattern and the overjet (see later).

The degree of crowding or spacing is now assessed along with the angulation (mesiodistal tip) and any rotations of the teeth. When all the teeth have erupted, the degree of crowding can be assessed visually by estimating the degree of overlap of each tooth at its contact points with the adjacent teeth. How far distally the lower canines would then have to move to enable the lower incisors to align without altering their labiolingual position can then be determined. In addition, an allowance has to be made for the contact points to align in the vertical plane. Thus the effect of the overbite and the curve of Spee has to be considered. A more accurate determination of the degree of crowding present, and which is applied to the whole arch, can be made by measuring the mesiodistal widths of all the teeth in one arch on a study model. The total of these measurements is then compared with the length of the whole arch when ignoring the presence of the crowding. This can be measured using a length of wire held on the study model (Fig. 5.4). This method will not, however, assess the crowding due to vertical contact point discrepancies or the curve of Spee.

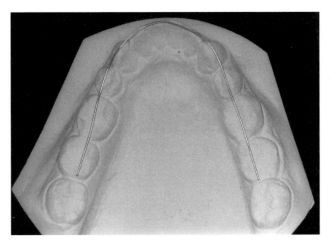

Fig. 5.4 Arch length can be determined using a piece of soft wire.

Generally, mild crowding in the lower arch is defined on being 1–2 mm per quadrant, moderate is up to 4 mm, and severe is greater than 4 mm. When such an assessment is made visually it is easy to over- or under-estimate the degree of crowding present. For example, 5.5 mm of crowding localized to one lower central incisor would totally exclude the tooth from the arch and quite rightly be classified as severe crowding. The same degree of crowding dispersed amongst several teeth might appear as mild crowding on first examination.

Although a description of the degree of crowding is very helpful, for many the description assumes more importance than how the crowding is distributed amongst the teeth being examined and consequently how easily it might be relieved. Using the examples above, severe localized crowding might be very easily treated by a single tooth extraction. The same degree of crowding spread over a greater number of teeth might indicate extraction of two premolar teeth within the arch and fixed appliance therapy. If difficulty is encountered in assigning the degree of crowding to a particular group, be it mild, moderate, or severe, generally it will have little effect on the final treatment plan. If in doubt, it is worth noting the approximate degree of crowding in millimetres. This can then be related to the degree of space that would be created by the extraction of a particular tooth. The choice of whether to extract or not, and if so which tooth to extract, will also be influenced by other factors which are dealt with in Chapter 10 (Treatment planning).

An assessment of the angulations of the labial segment teeth will aid in planning the most appropriate extraction pattern for the relief of crowding. This in turn will also help determine the type of orthodontic appliance required to achieve the desired tooth movement. For a spontaneous improvement in the alignment of teeth, those teeth adjacent to a planned extraction site should have their crowns angulated away from it (Fig. 5.5). Similarly, for simple tipping movements with a removable appliance the tooth to be moved must have a favourable crown angulation (Fig. 5.6). Where the crown is angulated towards a proposed extraction site a fixed appliance will be required to achieve the desired root movement into the extraction site, rather than crown movement. The degree of root movement necessary can be estimated both clinically and radiographically and will affect the anchorage and thus space requirements for the case.

Rotations are assessed and thus described by noting the part of the tooth that is furthest from the line of the arch (Fig. 5.7). As with differentiating between mild, moderate, and severe crowding,

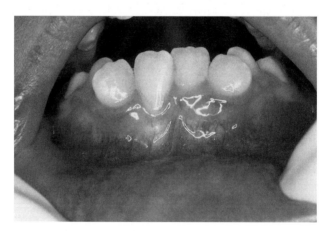

Fig. 5.5 For spontaneous tooth alignment, teeth adjacent to the extraction site should have their long axes angulated away from the potential extraction site as illustrated in this case where one of the lower incisors is being considered for extraction.

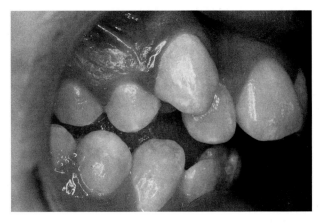

Fig. 5.6 A favourably mesially angulated canine which is suitable for retraction by tipping with a removable appliance.

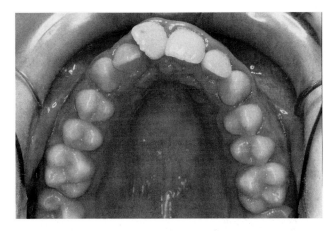

Fig. 5.7 This incisor tooth is described as being distolabially rotated, as this part of the tooth is furthest from the line of the arch.

more emphasis is often placed on describing a rotation in terms of the aspect of the tooth which is furthest from the line of the arch rather than recognizing how severely rotated a particular tooth is, or how many teeth are affected. What can also be difficult to determine is whether the rotation of a tooth is a manifestation of the degree of crowding, such that it would spontaneously align if space were provided, or whether it is a true, inherent rotation. In the latter case, the tooth would remain rotated even if space were provided. Generally a single tooth rotation is said to be readily correctable with a removable appliance whilst multiple rotations require fixed appliances for correction. In practise anything more than a 10–20° rotation, even of a single tooth, can be difficult to correct with a removable appliance and treatment with a fixed appliance is usually more expedient.

Assessment of malposed unerupted teeth has already been discussed. With erupted teeth, marked malpositions, such as a lingually placed lower incisor, need to be assessed in terms of how easily the tooth can be realigned within the arch. Root position as well as crown position is therefore important. A lingually positioned lower incisor may align spontaneously if provided with sufficient space or may require a simple tipping movement if the root apex is favourably within the line of the arch. If the root apex is also malposed the tooth may require bodily movement with a fixed appliance to achieve a good final position.

5.3 OVERJET

Overjet is defined as 'the horizontal distance between the labial surface of the tips of the upper incisors and the surface of the lower incisors'[5] This horizontal overlap is measured directly using a millimetre rule, for which a sterile 15 cm steel engineer's rule is the best instrument. With the teeth in centric occlusion the ruler is generally held parallel to the occlusal plane and the distance from the labial surface of a lower central incisor to the labial surface of the opposing upper central incisor is measured. Either the greatest overjet can be measured on the most prominent upper incisor, or the overjet on both upper centrals can be recorded. It is best to record the overjet at the most prominent part of an upper central incisor in the case of a rotated tooth, because an increased overjet is a good measure of the need for orthodontic treatment (see Chapter 7). It is, after all, the most prominent part of an upper incisor that is at greatest risk of traumatic injury. Although a measurement of overjet will indicate how far the incisal edges of the upper incisors must be moved in order to attain a normal overjet, in isolation it will not indicate how difficult it might be to achieve a class I incisor relationship with normal incisor inclinations. In the formulation of a treatment plan, overjet must therefore be considered in combination with skeletal pattern and the inclination of both the upper and lower incisor teeth. For example, a 10 mm overjet with proclined upper incisors on a class I skeletal base may be treated simply with removable appliances. The same 10 mm overjet, but where the upper incisors are of average inclination and where there is a severe class II skeletal base relationship, will require treatment involving fixed appliances in combination with orthognathic surgery. This is because the underlying anteroposterior skeletal discrepancy must be treated.

5.4 OVERBITE

This is the vertical overlap of the incisor teeth and can be described as average, increased, or decreased. An average overbite is where the upper incisors overlap the incisal third of the crowns of the lower incisors.

The overbite can then be described further as complete or incomplete, and if complete it will either be to tooth or to soft tissue. This soft tissue can either be the gingival margins palatal to the upper incisors or labial to the lower incisors, or it may be complete to the palate. In such cases it can lead to gingival recession or even cause soreness, in which case it is considered to be traumatic. If the overbite is markedly incomplete such that there is no vertical overlap, then it is described as an anterior open bite and the maximum extent of this can be measured using a millimetre rule. The assessment of overbite is important for the following reasons.

1. Can the overbite be accepted? A deep traumatic overbite is best treated while the patient is still growing, when correction may be relatively straightforward and before any long term periodontal damage occurs.

2. Is correction of the current overbite required for complete correction of another aspect of the malocclusion (e.g. overjet reduction)?

3. Does the overbite give a clue to possible aetiology of the maloc-
    clusion? For example, an anterior open bite might indicate an
    unfavourable skeletal or soft tissue pattern, or a persistent digit
    sucking habit. Commonly with digit sucking habits the anterior
    open bite is asymmetric (see Chapter 2). Symmetrical anterior
    open bites are more commonly seen when there is a vertical
    skeletal discrepancy (i.e. an increased anterior lower face
    height), or if the primary aetiological agent is an endogenous
    tongue thrust (see Chapter 2). An increased but just incom-
    plete overbite may indicate an adaptive swallowing pattern
    such as a tongue to lower lip swallow.

4. Is there, or will there be, sufficient overbite to maintain a stable
    incisor relationship at the end of treatment? For example, if an
    upper incisor is to be moved labially to correct an anterior
    crossbite in a class III incisor relationship, it is the presence of a
    positive overbite which will prevent subsequent relapse.

5.5 CENTRELINES

The upper and lower centre lines are assessed relative to each other
and to the midline of the face. Relative to each other it is usual to
record the centre line discrepancy between the upper and lower
arches in millimetres. With respect to the face the centre lines are
described as either being coincident with, or positioned to the right
or left of the facial midline, and this should be determined by
looking at the patient from above and behind. Once again measurement of a centre line discrepancy will not indicate ease of correction
on its own and needs to be considered in combination with the
angulations of the labial segment teeth. A centre line discrepancy
due to all the incisor teeth being angulated in one direction will be
easier to correct than if the incisors are of normal angulation. In the
former case simple tipping movements, perhaps with a removable
appliance, will facilitate centre line correction, while in the latter
case bodily movement with fixed appliances will be required.
Occasionally patients will notice their own centreline discrepancy,
but on the whole they will be unaware of any problem. From the
orthodontic point of view, centre lines are important if, at the end of
treatment, a full intercuspation of the canine and buccal segment
teeth is to be achieved with the correct incisor relationship.

5.6 BUCCAL SEGMENTS

As with the labial segment teeth the five features to be assessed in the buccal segments are:

(1) inclination

(2) crowding or spacing

(3) angulations

(4) rotations

(5) marked tooth malpositions.

The assessment of buccal segment tooth inclinations is important when a crossbite or scissors bite is present. The aim is to determine the degree of dento-alveolar compensation that is present and whether further orthodontic compensation would lead to the creation of a stable and functional result. This assessment is made by examining each arch with a view to determining the degree of curvature in the curve of Monson. Normally the palatal cusps of the upper buccal segment teeth appear slightly longer than the buccal cusps. If upper arch expansion is planned in order to deal with a posterior crossbite, it will be important that the upper buccal segment teeth are not already markedly buccally inclined, but are preferably palatally inclined (Fig. 5.8). In this way simple tipping movements of the teeth will achieve the desired expansion without an abnormal buccal inclination at the end of treatment.

Crowding, spacing, and tooth angulations within the buccal segments are assessed in a similar manner to that described for the labial segments. Rotations are again described in a similar manner to those in the labial segment, except the term 'buccal' is used instead of 'labial' in any description. For example, a distolabial rotation would be a distobuccal rotation in the buccal segment. The consequences of tooth rotations are different between the labial and buccal segments. Whereas rotated incisors and canines usually occupy less space within the arch and hence require the creation of space for their alignment, this is not the case with rotated buccal segment teeth. Rotated lower premolars will usually occupy the same amount of space as when aligned within the arch, whilst upper premolars and both upper and lower molars will generally occupy more space when rotated. Hence space will become available within the arch as they are derotated.

Markedly malposed teeth are assessed in the same manner as described previously.

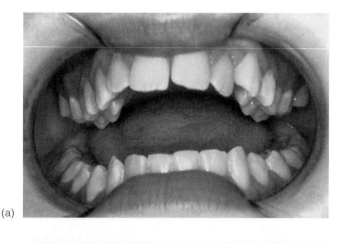

(a)

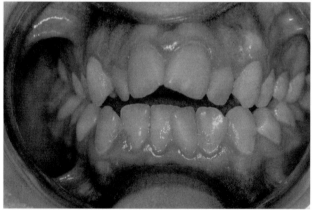

(b)

Fig. 5.8 Two intra-oral photographs are shown demonstrating the inclinations of the premolar teeth. (a) If the teeth are already flared, that is, inclined buccally as a result of dento-alveolar compensation, the upper arch cannot be expanded further using removable or simple fixed appliances to correct a crossbite. Notice that palatal cusps are evident. (b) In this case the teeth do not show the same dento-alveolar compensation and the arch can be expanded using a removable or fixed appliance to correct a buccal crossbite.

5.7 CROSSBITE AND SCISSORS BITE

In the normal occlusion, the anteroposterior relationship of the labial segment teeth is such that the lower incisors and canines occlude on the palatal surfaces of the upper labial segment teeth. Similarly, in the buccal segments the buccal cusps of the lower teeth occlude with the central fossae of the opposing upper buccal segment teeth. Crossbite or scissors bite occurs when this relationship is not present on one or more teeth.

A crossbite occurs when one or more upper labial segment teeth occlude palatal to the incisal edges or cusp tips of the corresponding lower arch teeth (Fig. 5.9). In the buccal segments a crossbite is seen when the buccal cusps of one or more upper teeth occlude in the central fossae of the lower buccal segment teeth. If a complete crossbite, as described, is not seen, then it is usual to describe, for example, a cusp to cusp relationship of upper and lower buccal segment teeth as a crossbite tendency. If one whole quadrant of buccal segment teeth are in crossbite this is described as a unilateral crossbite (Fig. 5.10). If both upper quadrants are involved a bilateral crossbite exists (Fig. 5.11). The three main aetiological agents involved in crossbite formation are skeletal pattern, habits, and crowding, as detailed below:

1. Skeletal pattern. Anteroposterior and transverse skeletal malrelationships can lead to the formation of anterior and posterior

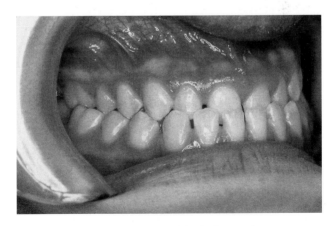

Fig. 5.9   An anterior crossbite affecting all the incisor teeth.

crossbites, respectively. Several teeth are usually involved and there is usually no displacement on any of the teeth on closing into centric occlusion (see later).

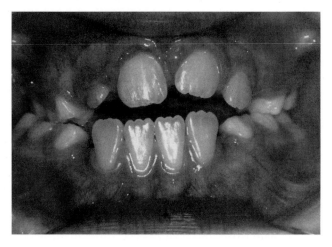

Fig. 5.10   A unilateral buccal crossbite affecting the maxillary first molar and deciduous molars on the right. However, deciduous molars should never be used to assess crossbites due to the nature of their exfoliation.

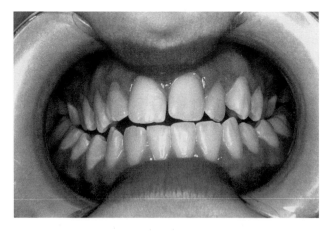

Fig. 5.11   A bilateral buccal crossbite.

2. Habits. A digit sucking habit usually leads to the formation of a unilateral crossbite with a displacement. The transverse skeletal relationship is correct, but the sucking habit leads to a contraction in the width of the upper arch. The mechanism of crossbite formation can be explained by visualizing the thumb in the vault of the palate. As a consequence the tongue moves to the floor of the mouth and opposing teeth in each arch are kept apart. During digit sucking the cheeks are drawn inwards against the teeth. If the teeth assume a position of balance between the cheeks and the tongue and yet the tongue is in the floor of the mouth there will be a decrease in the width of the upper arch, so that the upper arch width will approximate that of the lower arch. When the patient then attempts to close into centric occlusion, there will be a cusp to cusp relationship of the buccal segment teeth and the mandible will displace to one side on closing into maximum interdigitation, thereby producing a unilateral crossbite with a displacement (Fig. 5.12).

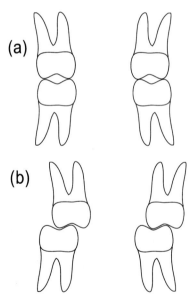

Fig. 5.12 A unilateral buccal crossbite in (a) the pre-displacement position and (b) maximum intercuspation, post-displacement.

3.   Crowding. When crowding causes the production of a crossbite
     it usually involves single teeth. Either lower arch teeth are labi-
     ally or buccally placed with respect to the rest of the arch, or
     upper arch teeth are palatally positioned.

A crossbite in isolation is not necessarily an indication for orthodontic treatment. However, when a crossbite is noted other factors
may determine whether it should be treated or accepted. A crossbite, with an associated displacement on closing into centric occlusion, is certainly a functional indication for orthodontic treatment.
Displacements can lead to unfavourable wear on teeth which can
then be difficult to restore. An example would be unfavourable
wear on an upper incisor tooth due to an anterior crossbite with a
displacement on the affected tooth (Fig. 5.13). It has also been suggested that displacements may have a limited role in the aetiology
of temporomandibular joint dysfunction (see Chapter 9).

Clinically, it can sometimes be difficult to determine whether a
crossbite has an associated mandibular displacement. The assessment is best done by asking the patient to relax, so that the clinician can then guide the mandible along its path of closure with the
mandibular condyles retruded within their fossae. When the first
occlusal contact is reached, the patient is then asked to continue
closing until they reach centric occlusion, or maximum intercuspation. At the same time the clinician must closely observe the path
of closure, not forgetting that a small anterior displacement (1.25
± 1 mm) into centric occlusion from the retruded position is quite
normal.[6] The importance of a displacement to the orthodontist is
that its presence will usually indicate that less tooth movement is
required for crossbite correction than when there is no displacement. In the case of anterior teeth, ideally the patient should be
able to achieve an edge to edge incisal relationship on the tooth or
teeth in crossbite. Moving affected teeth only 1 or 2 mm may then
lead to a complete correction of the crossbite, even though prior to
correction the reverse overjet may have measured much more than
this in centric occlusion. This subject is discussed further in
Chapter 6.

If there is no displacement associated with a crossbite, and certainly in the buccal segments where aesthetics are not a strong
consideration, it is perfectly acceptable to leave the crossbite
untreated. Indeed without a displacement, crossbite correction

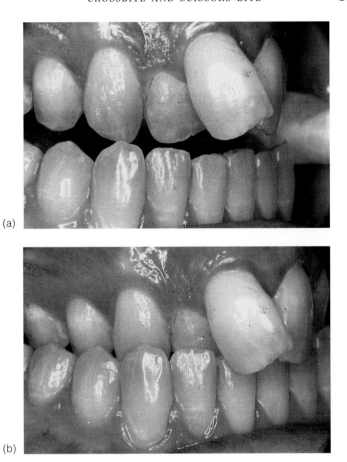

(a)

(b)

Fig. 5.13   Unfavourable wear on an upper lateral incisor and canine as a result of a crossbite (a). This is associated with an anterior and lateral displacement on closing into maximum intercuspation (b).

will often be very difficult and is unlikely to be stable, due usually to an underlying skeletal discrepancy. This is certainly the case with bilateral buccal crossbites. Crossbites can be subdivided as follows.

1.   Anterior – with or without a displacement. Usually, describe the teeth involved.

2. Posterior:

    (a) individual teeth – when less than a quadrant of teeth are involved, describe the teeth in crossbite and state whether there is a displacement or not;

    (b) unilateral – a whole quadrant of teeth is involved and there may or may not be an associated displacement on closing into centric occlusion;

    (c) bilateral – both quadrants of the arch are involved and usually without an associated displacement.

Another important feature to assess in relation to a crossbite is the vertical overlap, or overbite, of the teeth involved. This overlap will be a major determinant of post-treatment stability if the crossbite is to be corrected.

As discussed previously (p. 109), the inclination of teeth is another important consideration in treatment planning and this applies equally to the labial and buccal segment teeth. For example, if all the upper incisors are in crossbite, there is an anterior displacement on closing and a positive overbite – all of which might deem the crossbite as suitable for treatment – careful assessment needs to be made of both the skeletal pattern and the incisor inclinations. If there is a marked class III skeletal pattern, the upper incisors are already very proclined, and the lower incisors retroclined (dentoalveolar compensation), then orthodontic treatment alone is not recommended, even in the presence of a displacement. In such a case, treatment would result in unfavourable loading of the already proclined upper incisors and the interincisal angle would be further reduced. In addition, the final result may not fulfil the patient's expectations of aesthetics, since the principal cause of the crossbite may be the class III skeletal discrepancy, which requires surgical correction. On the other hand, a case with a similar initial reverse overjet, a positive overbite, a displacement on closing into centric occlusion, and where the upper incisors are retroclined, will be readily treatable with orthodontics. Indeed an upper removable appliance may be sufficient to procline the upper incisors over the bite, improving their inclination and correcting the crossbite with its associated displacement.

Scissors bites occur when upper arch teeth lie further buccally than their normal position. Like a crossbite it may affect either a few teeth or quadrants of teeth, and can once again be complete, where the upper tooth is entirely buccal to the corresponding lower arch tooth (see Chapter 2), or it may be buccal to a lesser degree and hence is described as a scissors bite tendency. Fortunately, unilateral and bilateral complete scissors bites are rarely found, and when they are, they are usually due to a marked skeletal discrepancy. A scissors bite tendency is, however, commonly observed in class II division 2 incisor relationships, localized to the upper first premolar regions (Fig. 5.14), and can be easily corrected as part of the overall treatment of the malocclusion.

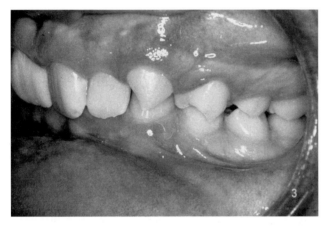

Fig. 5.14 A common finding in class II division 2 incisor relationships is a scissors bite localized to the first premolar teeth, the maxillary teeth occluding outside the mandibular teeth.

Summary of intra-oral examination

The following features are examined.
1. The teeth and supporting structures, in particular
    (a) presence
    (b) position
    (c) pathology
    (d) shape
    (e) size
    (f) developmental stage

continue on next page

Summary of intra-oral examination *(continued)*

2. Labial segments
   (a) inclination
   (b) crowding/spacing
   (c) angulations
   (d) rotations
   (e) malpositions
3. Overjet
4. Overbite
5. Centrelines
6. Buccal segments
   (a) inclination
   (b) crowding/spacing
   (c) angulations
   (d) rotations
   (e) malpositions
7. Crossbites and scissors bites

Objectives

1. Describe labial and buccal segment tooth relationships
2. Establish space requirements

REFERENCES

1. Bartlett, D. and Smith, B. G. N. (1994). The dental impact of eating disorders. *Dental Update*, **21**, 404–8.
2. Bartlett, D. and Smith, B. G. N. (1996). The dental relevance of gastro-oesophageal reflux: Part 2. *Dental Update*, **23**, 250–3.
3. Shaw, L. and Smith, A. (1994). Erosion in children: an increasing clinical problem? *Dental Update*, **21**, 103–7.
4. Polson, A. M. (1986). The relative importance of plaque and occlusion in periodontal disease. *Journal of Clinical Periodontology*, **13**, 923–7.
5. British Standards Institute (1983). Glossary of dental terms. B5 4492, BSI, London.
6. Posselt, U. (1952). Studies in the mobility of the human mandible. *Acta Odontologica Scandinavica*, **10** (Suppl.), 19–160.

6

Dynamic occlusion

The body is aware of each of its constituent parts, being able to relate them in three dimensions and this includes spatial awareness of the dentition and supporting tissues. The mechanism of recognizing spatial position and thereby coordinating muscle tone in particular, is known as proprioception. The mechanism consists of sensors (muscle spindles, Golgi tendon organs, Ruffini nerve endings, and free-ended fibres), afferent nerves, a central processing area of the central nervous system, efferent nerves (mostly motor nerves), and effectors, the striated muscles. When certain receptors are stimulated, the information is processed and physiological reflexes are activated.

Orthodontists are unique in their ability to change the dentition, altering the position of the teeth from that acquired during the development of the occlusion. This can then modify the proprioceptive input from the teeth, jaws, and soft tissues. Fortunately the majority of orthodontic treatment is carried out in patients who have an adaptive potential, capable of remodelling both bony tissues and adapting neural systems, to the new post-treatment position. It is also clear that the ability to accommodate neurophysiological change decreases with age and that stepping beyond 'the envelope of adaptation' may lead to disorders/pathophysiology. This is especially true of the temporomandibular joint, capable of some internal remodelling, yet also capable of producing symptoms and signs which are distressing to both the patient and the operator. The symptoms in such cases are so imprecise as to give imperfect 'non-scientific' methodologies credence, with a very diffuse boundary between placebo effects and realistic treatment results. As a consequence many 'snake-oil salesmen' peddle their wares with no basis in fact. Examination of the functioning teeth and jaws is therefore important before planning and then carrying out orthodontic treatment. This is especially so if a patient presents with temporomandibular joint symptoms or pain.

6.1 CLINICAL EXAMINATION

It is fairly simple to observe the opening and closing of the mandible from rest to maximum intercuspation. Observing the patient either directly from in front, or from above and behind, will enable any deviations of mandibular movement from the midline to be readily recognized. Subsequent examination of the joints may be undertaken by bilateral palpation as the mouth opens and closes (Fig. 6.1). Use of a stereo-stethoscope to listen to any joint sounds or crepitus will enable the more subtle disorders of function to be identified. Occasional sounds such as clicks may also be audible without the aid of such instruments. Following the extra-oral palpation it is often necessary to examine the major muscles of mastication to establish whether they are tender to palpation. A tender

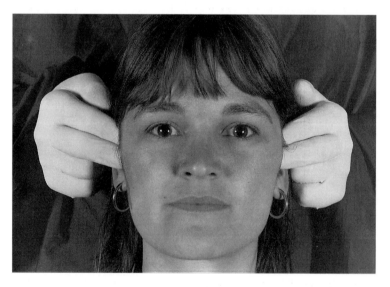

Fig. 6.1 Bilateral palpation of the skin overlying the temporomandibular joints. The patient is asked to open and close in a controlled manner and any changes from a smooth movement are noted.

tender muscle indicates a build up of the products of inflammation as a result of overloading, for example following excessive bruxism or clenching. It can be a straightforward process identifying the precipitating factors of temporomandibular joint dysfunction such as displacements on closing into centric occlusion, but in most instances the aetiology is unknown.

During orthodontic diagnosis, when examining occlusal relationships, it is important that the patient is assessed with the mandibular condyles retruded in the correct position within the glenoid fossae. Incorrect assessment can lead to many potential problems during treatment. For example, failing to diagnose an anterior displacement of the mandible, as a consequence of a premature tooth contact on an instanding upper incisor, may lead to the inaccurate assessment of the skeletal pattern. If the skeletal pattern is assessed as class I when it is in fact class II, the wrong teeth may be extracted for the relief of crowding and correction of the malocclusion. Once treatment is under way and the anterior displacement of the mandible is corrected, the overjet will be seen to increase. If the maxillary second premolars had been extracted for the relief of crowding, the space created may now appear insufficient to align the teeth and reduce the now apparently increased overjet. That is, there is insufficient anchorage and extraction of the upper first premolars would have been more appropriate.

Sometimes it is not possible to identify a causative premature contact and minor displacement in a standard 'orthodontic' examination and it may be necessary to resort to the use of specific jigs/cotton wool rolls as adjuncts in establishing the correct 'centric relation' prior to determining whether or not there is a premature contact. The specific steps are outlined in textbooks of conservative dentistry,[1] but essentially consists of the following:

1. Ask the patient to lie supine and with the chin pointing upwards.
2. Stabilize the head, possibly between the operator's abdomen and forearm.
3. Place four fingers on each side of the mandible, with the thumbs placed above the soft tissue chin (Fig. 6.2).
4. Apply gentle pressure to open and close the mandible in no more than 1–2 mm movements.
5. Confirm the position of centric relation by applying firm pressure upwards on the mandible while resisting this with the thumbs.

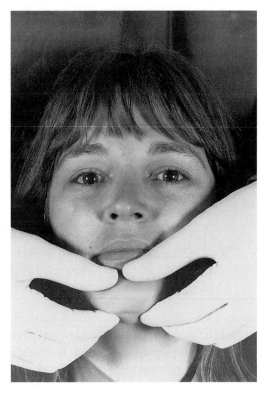

Fig. 6.2   In order to elicit a displacement it is necessary to overcome any habitual muscle activity. By careful manipulation of the mandible (see text for details) it is feasible to demonstrate a displacement in the majority of cases where one exists and is hidden by inherent muscle behaviour.

6.   Normally, the mandible should not translate off its hinge axis of closure (i.e. no lateral or posterior slides of the condylar head will occur), although a small anterior slide into maximum inter-cuspation is perfectly normal.

6.2 FUNCTIONAL OCCLUSION

Guidance of the mandible into its working and non-working paths of closure should be considered both anteroposteriorly and laterally.

Abnormal occlusal contacts in function can lead to unfavourable and sometimes excessive occlusal loading of the teeth. Typically it leads to a 'jiggling' type of loading during mastication. Such loading will lead to remodelling within the periodontium and surrounding alveolar bone. Whereas the healthy periodontium may be able to withstand this, if it should occur in combination with inflammatory disease it can cause rapid gingival detachment and bony degeneration, which will inevitably compromise long-term dental health.

Clearly when examining mandibular movement it is therefore important to be sure of the working and non-working contacts of the dynamic, functioning occlusion (see Glossary). In general two types of dental guidance can be found in lateral movements of the mandible, depending on the teeth guiding the disclusion (see Glossary). These are canine guidance and group function. Anterior guidance occurs on the incisor teeth.

6.2.1 Canine guidance

When moving from the position of maximum intercuspation to a position lateral to this, the canines cause the mandible to disclude away from the maxilla on the working side. On the side away from the lateral excursion (i.e. the non-working side), there should be no contacts. This is referred to as a mutually protected occlusion in which the posterior teeth make contact in centric occlusion only. In protrusion the incisors are the only teeth that are in contact. In this arrangement all lateral forces are resisted by the canines.

The anatomy of the canine crown prevents the development of any significant lateral forces and the overall function tends to be lateral in nature. Furthermore, the good crown–root ratio of the canine, as well as being situated in some of the denser bone of the maxilla, favours the canine as a tooth capable of withstanding this loading.

6.2.2 Group function

When the mandible moves laterally from centric occlusion, all posterior teeth on the working side make contact in harmony. As the mandible moves further laterally so the molars slowly disclude, starting with the most posterior molar which has the shortest contact stroke and finishing with the canine with the longest contact. On the non-working side there should be no contacts.

6.2.3 Anterior guidance

Anterior guidance describes the movement of the mandible from the position of maximum intercuspation to an edge to edge incisal relationship (assuming a class I incisor relationship). The lower incisor edges move down the palatal surfaces of the maxillary incisors and, in so doing, prevent any posterior working contacts. Problems with anterior guidance are less frequent than with lateral functional movements.

6.3 MANDIBULAR PATHS OF OPENING AND CLOSURE

6.3.1 Rest position

The starting position of the mandible in relation to the maxilla is referred to as the rest position. There are many factors which control the actual position of the mandible in space, including a close association with head posture and also the general cerebral activity of the patient. The rest position is extremely variable, showing intra- and inter-individual characteristics, although the extremes of this variation are limited in dimension. In general the circum-mandibular muscles, both masticatory and facial, are relaxed and the condyles are in a retruded unloaded or unstrained position. The distance between the upper and lower dentition is known as the freeway space and is commonly 4–5 mm in the premolar region.

The position of the mandible in this rest position is referred to as 'centric relation' which refers to a positional relationship of the temporomandibular joints (i.e. the condyles in the glenoid fossae). It also infers an axial element, in that for the mandible to open or close there is a rotational movement around a fixed axis. A fuller anatomical definition is that 'centric relation' exists when the properly aligned condyle and disc structures are in the most superior position against the joint eminence irrespective of the vertical dimension or dental position. This is in contrast to the term 'centric occlusion' when the teeth take up the position of maximum intercuspation. This can occur irrespective of the position of the disc and condylar head. Occlusal treatment is often described as successful when the two positions are identical with respect to the positioning of the disc/condyle apparatus, that is, the most posterion superior position in the glenoid fossae.

6.3.2 Habit postures

In the majority of the population the mandible can easily be moved
to the rest position. In some severe malocclusions the patients may
habitually posture the mandible downwards and forwards mainly to
camouflage the underlying dental/skeletal problem. Alternatively,
this position is assumed subconsciously in an attempt to achieve a
lip to lip anterior oral seal (see below). Other postures include the
increased freeway space in association with a low Frankfort–
mandibular planes angle, typical of a class II division 2 incisor relationship. Finally, in class III incisor relationships, a patient may
habitually posture the mandible anteriorly in order to prevent excessive loading of the incisors, which might otherwise be in an edge to
edge relationship, and to reduce the freeway space to a physiolo-
gically accepted range.

6.3.3 Path of closure

Ideally the mandible will move from the rest position to the position
of maximum intercuspation, 2 to 3 mm, by a simple hinge type
movement on its fixed condylar axis. Two variations are found
from this.

1. The mandible is held in a postured position as outlined above
    but is found to be in the correct centric relationship on closure.
    This is known as a deviation of the mandible and is defined as
    closure into centric occlusion from a postured position.

2. When the mandible moves from the rest position to centric
    occlusion, a contact with one or more teeth (premature
    contact) might occur. This causes the mandible to deviate from
    its simple hinge movement and this is known as a displacement.
    A displacement is defined as closure into centric occlusion fol-
    lowing a premature contact with a movement of the mandible
    off its ideal hinge axis. The mandible may move backwards (as
    in class II division 2 type incisor relationships, especially if there
    has been a loss of posterior teeth), forwards (as with instanding
    upper incisors and some class III incisor relationships), or later-
    ally (unilateral crossbites as a result of thumb sucking).

It is essential to distinguish between deviations and displacements, as the treatment will differ. Deviations will not normally be

linked with or give rise to pain, faceting of the teeth, or periodontal breakdown, whereas displacements may, in the long term, be associated with all of these problems.

Mandibular deviations are associated with habit postures. In a class II division 1 case, with the mandible in the habit position, the interocclusal clearance is often increased and the condyles are forward in the glenoid fossae. The path of closure is usually upwards and backwards, but when the teeth are in occlusion the condyles are in a normal position in the glenoid fossae. One aspect to consider with these types of deviations is that orthodontic treatment using some form of myofunctional appliance may be very complex. The existence of the habit may prevent the neuromuscular reflexes from provoking the muscle contraction which in turn provides the force for orthodontic movement and correction of the malocclusion.

The presence of a deviation is not a functional indication for performing orthodontic treatment. However, by treating the malocclusion, the deviation should also be eliminated.

Unlike a deviation, a displacement is associated with a premature occlusal contact prior to the patient reaching a position of maximum intercuspation. Displacements are frequently long-standing, having developed during eruption of the teeth. In some instances the displacement is established in the deciduous dentition, and as the permanent teeth erupt, they too are guided by occlusal forces into a crossbite that perpetuates the displacement. However, care is needed to interpret a crossbite in the deciduous dentition. Not only do deciduous teeth undergo occlusal wear, which can make assessment of occlusal relationships difficult, but upper deciduous molars often move slightly palatally as their permanent successors erupt.

Displacements can also arise later in life due to uncontrolled drifting of the teeth, either as a consequence of unplanned extractions or periodontal breakdown. For example, loss of posterior support following extractions can lead to a posterior displacement with overclosure, especially in class II division 2 cases. Periodontal disease is still the commonest cause of tooth loss, especially posterior teeth.

It is important to recognize that once a malocclusion has become established, considerable adjustment and tooth movement may be required to eliminate a displacement and subsequently modify the neuromuscular pathways. It is therefore prudent to correct occlusal disharmonies that are associated with mandibular displacements at the earliest possible opportunity and preferably during development of the occlusion. This is one of the rare indications for early treatment, but should not be seen as a recommendation that all treatment should be started at an early stage.

Lateral displacements are frequently associated with unilateral crossbites. If the maxillary and mandibular arches are of similar widths, a lateral displacement of the mandible is necessary to obtain a position of maximum intercuspation and a unilateral crossbite is produced (see Chapter 5). Lateral displacements are not associated with an increased interocclusal clearance nor with overclosure of the mandible. However, in a proportion of cases, muscle pain/temporomandibular dysfunction will develop and will be alleviated only on elimination of the displacement. The evidence linking displacements with temporomandibular joint dysfunction is extremely equivocal (see Chapter 9).

The presence of a unilateral crossbite, particularly where the centrelines are not coincident, should indicate to the clinician that a lateral displacement may be present. This can be confirmed as outlined previously. It is helpful to note the relationship of the centrelines both with the mandible at rest and in centric occlusion. Clearly the occlusal interference should be corrected. If there is a unilateral crossbite, symmetrical expansion of the upper arch with an orthodontic appliance is indicated. It should be noted, however, that not all unilateral crossbites are associated with lateral displacement of the mandible as there may be a true asymmetry of the upper or lower arch. If there is no displacement, the crossbite will give rise to no functional disability and correction may not be indicated.

Anteroposterior displacements may arise through premature contacts in the incisor region or as previously discussed, in class II division 2 incisor relationships with loss of posterior teeth. In such cases there is sometimes over-closure of the mandible into centric occlusion. This is especially so in class III incisor relationships where all four incisors are in crossbite. Whenever there are instanding upper incisors it is important to identify any anterior displacement as not only will it affect the function of the masticatory apparatus but also the long-term health of the teeth. It will also modify treatment planning, such as extraction choice.

Equally important is that a unilateral crossbite associated with a displacement can be very simple to treat. Due to the development of such a condition, the actual amount of expansion required is very little, the molars meeting in a cusp to cusp relationship. Thus the

maxillary dentition is not significantly narrower than the mandibular; the displacement makes it appear more complex.

6.3.4 The use of articulators

It is possible to reproduce a complete set of functioning records of the
patient's occlusion using articulators. They are available in many
forms, the commonest of which is the simple hinge articulator. This
usefully replicates the first 'normal' movements of the mandible (i.e.
a simple hinge axis with its centre at the condylar axis), assisting in
the construction of bite platforms and functional appliances. This can
greatly reduce the chair-side time when fitting such appliances. A
less commonly used articulator is the fully adjustable type, capable of
simulating a greater range of condylar movement. These articulators are often used in conjunction with a facebow recording in order
to relate the teeth to the facial skeleton. Use of such specialist equipment requires an appropriate level of technical laboratory support if
the articulated study casts are to be of clinical use. The main indications for using an adjustable articulator are:

(1) surgical and occlusal planning in cases requiring orthognathic
surgery; or

(2) occlusal assessment in any patient with persistent temporomandibular joint symptoms/signs.

Summary of dynamic occlusion

1. Extra-oral examination:
    Assessment, where present, of mandibular deviations, temporo-
    mandibular joint sounds, and palpable crepitus. Masticatory
    muscles can be palpated for signs of tenderness.
2. Intra-oral examination: Functional occlusion:
    (a) canine guidance
    (b) group function
    (c) anterior guidance
3. Mandibular paths of opening and closure:
    (a) rest position
    (b) habit postures
    (c) path of closure – displacements and deviations

Objectives

1. Outline the types of dental guidance found during movements of the mandible
2. Define displacement and deviation

REFERENCES

1. Dawson, P. E. (1989). *Evaluation, diagnosis and treatment of occlusal problems*, (2nd edn). C. V. Mosby, Missouri.

7

Health considerations

In the determination of an orthodontic treatment plan, health, and in particular dental health, is a most important consideration. Along with improved oral function and improved aesthetics, health gain is one of the three principal reasons for performing orthodontic treatment. An assessment of dental health in terms of past history, and present and possible future status therefore needs to be made as part of the diagnostic process. Each presenting malocclusion can usually be treated in different ways but whatever the chosen treatment plan, it is important that health is improved, not compromised, as a result of the orthodontic treatment. Health considerations will therefore assist in the setting of realistic treatment objectives and thus help determine the most appropriate treatment plan for a particular patient. Important health considerations are dental caries, periodontal disease, prevention of traumatic injury, and psychosocial well-being. These will now be considered in more detail.

7.1 DENTAL CARIES

In examining the teeth for caries, the clinician needs to assess the presence of active caries; its previous influence on the dentition and any future effect. This may then modify the decision as to whether to treat the malocclusion or not.

7.1.1 Past caries experience

The number and size of any restorations will have an obvious bearing on the orthodontic treatment plan. Teeth with large and particularly multi-surface restorations, or where the enamel surrounding a restoration is very thin, are likely to have an unfavourable prognosis. Where possible these should be incorporated into any extraction regimen. Sometimes this will increase treatment complexity, and might mean fixed rather than removable appliances have to be used. Alternatively, headgear may be necessary to reinforce anchorage when otherwise the case could have been managed with extractions alone. An example of such a case might be a class II division 1 incisor relationship on a class I skeletal base requiring the loss of all four first premolars and the use of an upper removable appliance to complete the treatment. If one or more of the upper second premolars is heavily restored, the latter tooth rather than the first premolar will have to be extracted. This will usually necessitate the use of fixed appliances to create a good contact between the first premolar and first permanent molar, and may also mean headgear will be required to reinforce the anchorage. Root-treated teeth should also be included in any extraction regimen where possible, although root treatment itself is not a contraindication to orthodontic tooth movement.[1]

Past caries experience is often a good indicator of an increased caries risk[2] and a careful examination should be made for active caries, especially in the heavily restored dentition.

7.1.2 Present active caries

An essential part of the examination procedure is the diagnosis of active caries. Extraction of a healthy tooth when there is active caries elsewhere in the mouth is best avoided. Visual examination, under good illumination and after drying the teeth, will assist in diagnosis, but even under ideal laboratory conditions carious lesions which are into dentine can easily be missed.[3] In the case of occlusal caries, probing is not recommended due to poor reliability and the risk of damage to the enamel of the fissure. It has been suggested that detection of occlusal caries has become more difficult since the advent of fluoride toothpaste.[4] This is due to enamel remineralization masking the underlying dentine caries until the lesion is very large. Whereas this large dentine lesion will often be visible on a dental panoramic tomogram (DPT), early lesions which have only just progressed into dentine may not be visible. Both interstitial and occlusal caries may be detectable on bitewing radiographs and consideration should therefore be given to obtaining such radiographs prior to commencing orthodontic treatment, especially where fixed orthodontic appliances are to be used. Should such radiographs be required subsequent to starting fixed appliance therapy, it will necessitate removal and then refitting of the appliance. If there is doubt as to the presence of caries, the opinion of the patient's general dental practitioner should be sought and the tooth in question investigated further. Written confirmation as to the prognosis and condition of the tooth then needs to be obtained before an orthodontic treatment plan is finalized.

7.1.3 Caries prevention

There is little evidence to suggest that occlusal irregularity has a significant effect on the incidence of dental caries. This is perhaps not surprising as caries is a multifactorial disease most commonly affecting the occlusal surfaces of teeth.[5] In a study of 11–12 year old children[6] it was demonstrated that irregular teeth accumulate more plaque than well aligned teeth. From this it might be expected that the incidence of caries would be greater in those individuals with irregular teeth, since a relationship between plaque control and smooth surface caries has been previously reported.[7,8] No such relationship, however, was found between occlusal irregularity and either gingivitis or dental caries in the 11–12 year old individuals examined in that study. Caries prevention cannot therefore be considered an indication for performing orthodontic treatment in most patients. In certain circumstances, orthodontic correction of particular tooth malpositions can assist in caries prevention, or perhaps permit the easier restoration of a tooth should a carious lesion develop at a later date. An example of this would be a mesio-angularly impacted lower second molar. Uprighting the tooth may facilitate the placement of a fissure sealant as a preventive measure, or if occlusal caries is already present, it may permit the placement of an adequate restoration.

7.2 PERIODONTAL DISEASE

Examination of the periodontal tissues in an orthodontic patient will to some extent be determined by the age of the patient and the presenting complaint. Most orthodontic patients are in their early teens and as a consequence are likely to have little in the way of chronic periodontal disease with associated loss of attachment. However, the presence of gingivitis in children is almost universal, with up to 80 per cent of children under 12 years of age and almost 100 per cent of children by 14 years of age having some areas of gingival inflammation.[9] The fact that gingivitis is so common does not make it acceptable and orthodontic treatment should not be instigated until the disease has been brought under control. The primary aetiological agent in periodontal disease is dental plaque and a good standard of oral hygiene must be achieved if orthodontic treatment is to be performed.[10] Gingival inflammation cannot be resolved by extra vigilant brushing on the day of the orthodontic examination. The inflammation present is a measure of the patient's response to plaque. Therefore, assessment of the gingival condition is a more meaningful and relevant criterion upon which to base a patient's suitability for orthodontic treatment. A visual examination of the gingivae will usually permit a diagnosis of gingivitis to be made. If a patient presents with chronic marginal gingivitis at the initial examination and is to go through a regimen of oral hygiene instruction then the presence or absence of bleeding can be monitored along with gingival appearance by using a bleeding index, that is, the proportion of sites which bleed on gentle probing.[11] Ideally no areas of gingival inflammation, either acute or chronic, should be present at the commencement of orthodontic treatment since it is known that fixed orthodontic appliances can lead to gingival inflammation even in patients with apparently good oral hygiene.[12] It is inevitably made worse when the standard of oral hygiene is poor. Although this gingival inflammation will subside within a few weeks of cessation of orthodontic treatment when a good standard of oral hygiene is maintained, irreversible damage may occur to the teeth and supporting structures during treatment. At the enamel surface, decalcification may lead to white spot formation or even cavitation. In the case of the periodontal tissues it is known that up to 46 per cent of 15 year old children may exhibit early signs of periodontal destruction.[13] The concern is that this might be compounded by the alveolar bone remodelling that is known to take place during orthodontic fixed appliance therapy, even in the presence of good oral hygiene.[14] If gingivitis is still present despite repeated oral hygiene instruction then the malocclusion must either be accepted or a less complex approach contemplated. This may mean an extraction-only approach, with very limited treatment objectives, or perhaps simple removable appliance therapy where the appliance can be removed for cleaning. In such cases the risks involved in orthodontic treatment must be considered against the benefits, ranging from the simplest to the most complex form of treatment.

For example, consider two patients with only fair oral hygiene and who have a few areas of chronic gingivitis. One has a class I incisor relationship with mild crowding and the other a class II division 1 incisor relationship with a 12 mm overjet. In the former example the only indication for treatment might be aesthetic improvement, and treatment may only be deemed possible by the loss of a second premolar in each quadrant of the mouth and the use of upper and lower fixed appliances. Any other form of treatment such as simple removable appliance therapy would provide little, if any, improvement. In the second, class II division 1 case, the indications for treatment are likely to be threefold, namely improvement in aesthetics, prevention of trauma to the upper incisors, and also prevention of gingival drying in the same region.[15] This case might also require treatment with fixed appliances. A risk/benefit analysis of the two case examples would suggest the benefits of treatment may well outweigh the risks in the class II division 1 case, but are unlikely to do so in the class I case. If treatment with fixed appliances is still felt to entail too much risk in the class II division 1 case, then treatment with removable appliances, if possible, might be considered to be acceptable in terms of the risk/benefit analysis.

With adult patients a simple and rapid assessment of periodontal status is required prior to treatment planning and this can be done using the BSP/CPITN screening system[16] (British Society of Periodontology/community periodontal index of treatment needs). This entails dividing the mouth into sextants and measuring probing depths with a World Health Organization (WHO) periodontal probe at a minimum of six sites around each of the teeth. The highest score for each sextant is then recorded. The probe (Fig. 7.1) has a coloured band extending from 3.5 to 5.5 mm and should be used with a recommended probing force of 20–25 g. Scoring is as follows.

Code 4: Coloured band disappears into pocket, indicating a probing depth of ≥ 6 mm.

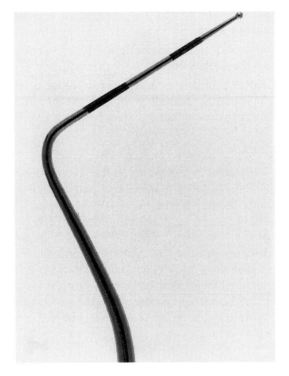

Fig. 7.1 The CPITN probe has a coloured band extending from 3.5 to 5.5 mm.

Code 3: Coloured band remains partly visible in deepest pocket of sextant.

Code 2: Coloured band remains entirely visible but calculus or defective restoration margin detected supra- or subgingivally.

Code 1: Coloured band remains entirely visible in the deepest pocket but bleeding is present.

Code 0: Healthy gingival tissue with no bleeding on probing.

Code *: Denotes two features, either furcation involvement or recession, plus probing depth totalling 7 mm or more.

The recommended treatment, once the scores have been determined, is given below.[17]

Code 0: No treatment required.

Code 1: Oral hygiene instruction and prophylaxis.

Code 2: Treat as code 1 with the addition of supra- and sub-gingival scaling.

Code 3: Treat as code 2, but follow up yearly with detailed probing depth measurement.

Code 4: Extensive periodontal assessment from the outset of treatment including detailed probing depth measurement and radiographic examination. Treatment will be as code 3 but is also likely to include root planing and periodontal surgery.

Care must be taken in the interpretation of the scores obtained using the BSP/CPITN screen in adolescent patients due to the likely presence of false pocketing. If the screen is used in such patients it is suggested that only six teeth are examined, namely the first permanent molars, and the upper right and lower left central incisors. This is because they are the first permanent teeth to erupt and are therefore less likely to show false pocketing and more likely to show evidence of periodontal disease. In cases of juvenile periodontitis it is also these teeth that commonly show the earliest evidence of disease. In children between 7 and 11 years of age the BSP/CPITN screen can again be used.

Although interstitial alveolar bone loss due to periodontal disease is most readily detected using bitewing or periapical radiographs, a DPT is routinely taken to aid orthodontic diagnosis and may provide a useful screening, particularly for younger patients. It does, however, have a tendency to underestimate minor marginal bone loss and overestimate major bone loss.

7.3 ORTHODONTIC/PERIODONTIC CONSIDERATIONS

Although it is necessary to perform a risk/benefit analysis prior to orthodontic treatment for patients with less than ideal standards of oral hygiene, generally only when the necessary periodontal treatment has been performed and disease brought under control can orthodontic treatment be planned. Teeth which have undergone extensive loss of alveolar support have a number of important characteristics relevant to orthodontic treatment, namely:

(1) they are easily and quickly moved using an orthodontic appliance;

(2) they are not good at providing anchorage for the movement of other teeth;

(3) they have a greater tendency to return to their pretreatment position following orthodontic treatment, under the influence of factors such as the soft tissues. For this reason, teeth whose position has been corrected following periodontal drifting must have their position retained on an indefinite basis. They can either be retained permanently using a rigid metal retainer such as a Rochette or Maryland splint, by conventional fixed bridgework, or by using a flexible bonded retainer made from multistrand orthodontic wire.[18] Woven Kevlar® is now also available for this purpose. Alternatively the patient may wear a removable retainer at night for the rest of their life.

Occasionally a child presents in the mixed dentition with marked gingival recession on the labial aspect of one crowded lower permanent incisor tooth. The alveolar bone overlying a labially positioned root may be very thin and may even show some signs of a fenestration or dehiscence. As a consequence, inflammation due to poor oral hygiene can lead to rapid gingival recession. In such instances, consideration can be given to the extraction of the lower deciduous canines in order to relocate the crowding in the lower labial segment and permit the labially positioned tooth to move lingually, closer to the line of the dental arch. In this way it is anticipated that the risk of further recession will be reduced when combined with adequate oral hygiene measures. This labial positioning is sometimes associated with a crossbite involving the opposing upper incisor tooth. Interceptive correction of the crossbite is indicated to remove the traumatic occlusion and prevent further gingival recession on the labially positioned lower incisor. Indeed, once corrected it has been shown that the degree of measured recession improves over the following year even after any improvement in oral hygiene standards has been taken into account.[19] In the permanent dentition, when perhaps definitive fixed appliance therapy is being performed, it will be important either to actively realign a labially positioned tooth into a more lingual position, or at least to ensure that during alignment of the lower incisors they are not proclined, even transiently, during the early stages of treatment. Such transient proclination will often occur during the early initial alignment phase with fixed orthodontic appliances, even in cases where premolar extractions have been carried out. In order to prevent this it may be necessary to begin treatment without bonding brackets to the lower incisor teeth and to retract the lower canines first. Space can thereby be created to allow some spontaneous improvement in the lower incisor position before finally actively aligning the incisors with the appliance. The presence of such recession would favour extractions for the relief of crowding when it is felt the case could be treated by either an extraction or non-extraction approach.

Another appliance which commonly causes proclination of the lower incisor teeth, often as an unwanted effect, is the functional appliance used for the treatment of class II division 1 incisor relationships. It is usual to try to reduce the likelihood of this proclination in the design of the appliance by not having the appliance make contact with the lower incisor teeth. The most important feature to correct, however, is the oral hygiene and hence gingival inflammation at the commencement of treatment and for this to be maintained throughout the course of treatment and beyond.

Deep traumatic overbites which are complete to the palatal gingivae of the upper incisors or the labial gingivae of the lower incisors are most detrimental to dental health in the presence of poor oral hygiene (see Chapter 2). Early diagnosis of such overbites is important in order to prevent damage to the gingivae and because treatment in the growing child is usually quite straightforward. Once a patient reaches adulthood and facial growth has all but ceased, the only means of treatment might be via a surgical correction of the malocclusion using a combined orthodontic and orthognathic approach.

7.4 TRAUMATIC INJURIES TO THE TEETH

The incidence of incisal trauma is reported to be between 4.2 and 25 per cent[20–22] with most injuries occurring between 8 and 11 years of age.[23] Of these, most occur in class II division 1 incisor relationships where the risk of injury is five times greater than in a case with a normal incisor relationship and hence normal overjet. Indeed, the greater the overjet the more teeth are usually injured.[24] Once an overjet reaches 10 mm, for boys in particular, there is a 1 in 4 chance of traumatic injury to the incisors by the age of 13 years.[25] A relationship has also been found between lip incompetence and incisal trauma.[26] Orthodontic correction of an increased overjet in children is therefore not only likely to prevent an unpleasant traumatic episode, but will also obviate the need for extensive and repeated crown and bridgework over the remainder of a patient's lifetime. However, overjet reduction performed during the mixed dentition suffers three potential disadvantages.

1. Overjet reduction will form the initial stage of treatment, but definitive treatment of the whole occlusion will not be possible until the permanent dentition has developed. Treatment will therefore be protracted.

2. Due to the protracted nature of the treatment, patient motivation and cooperation may be a problem following overjet reduction.

3. Care must be taken to assess the position of the unerupted upper permanent canines relative to the roots of the upper incisors. The clinical assessment should be supplemented by a radiographic examination utilizing the parallax technique (see Chapter 8). Sometimes it will not be possible to reduce the overjet until the canines have erupted. This is due to the risk of tipping the upper lateral incisor roots into the unerupted canine crowns, thereby inducing root resorption in the former. In such a case treatment should be deferred and the patient advised to wear a mouthguard during contact sports and other high risk pastimes such as cycling and roller-skating.

In cases where a class II skeletal malrelationship requires correction, treatment with a functional appliance can be started during the late mixed dentition in order to take advantage of facial growth during the pubertal growth spurt. Not all of the overjet reduction will necessarily be achieved by tipping of the upper incisors and the risk to the upper lateral incisor roots from the unerupted canine crowns will therefore hopefully be lower. In all cases the risk of upper lateral incisor root resorption from the unerupted canines must be weighed against the advantages of early treatment of the malocclusion. The need to correct the malocclusion at a time of rapid facial growth, without which orthodontic treatment alone may not be possible due to the severity of the underlying skeletal malrelationship, is an example where early treatment would be of great benefit. Similarly, if a patient has suffered repeated trauma to the upper incisors, the advantages of treatment preventing further such episodes may greatly outweigh the aforementioned disadvantages to early treatment of the increased overjet. This is a further example of a risk/benefit analysis in orthodontic diagnosis and treatment planning.

7.5 PSYCHOSOCIAL WELL-BEING

The presence of a malocclusion may have two psychological effects. The first will be via the response of others to the deformity, and the second will be the effect the deformity has on a person's own sense of well-being and self-esteem. Investigations into the psychological effects of dentofacial deformity have found that children with a malocclusion are much more susceptible to teasing by their peers.[27] Indeed, adults recalling their malocclusions from some 15 years previously stated that traits such as increased overjet, increased overbite, and crowding, especially of the upper incisors, lead to teasing and the individuals being unhappy with their appearance.[28] However, the distress caused by such disfigurement is not necessarily directly proportional to anatomic severity.[29] It has been stated that the most severely disfigured could anticipate a consistently negative response from others, while those with less severe disfigurement such as a retrognathic mandible or protruding upper incisors did not receive a consistent response. Such unpredictable responses produce anxiety and can have strongly deleterious effects.[30] Attractive persons, without such deformities, are regarded as being more popular[31,32] and are perceived as having greater intelligence[33,34] and educational potential.[35]

7.6 DETERMINING THE NEED FOR ORTHODONTIC TREATMENT

In recent years there has been a move towards prioritizing treatment towards those malocclusions which would benefit the most from correction. This has been brought about partly by financial constraints within publicly funded health systems and also the shortage of orthodontic manpower able to cope with the ever increasing demand for high quality orthodontic treatment. In particular there has been a move by health authorities, who purchase orthodontics on behalf of the general public, only to fund treatments in which there is going to be a demonstrable health gain. An index of need for treatment has been used by the Swedish Health Board for a number of years in order to set priorities in the allocation of resources. More recently this has been refined to give the index of orthodontic treatment need (IOTN)[36] which is subdivided into two parts, a dental health component (DHC) and an aesthetic component (AC). Like the original, the dental health component has five dental health categories as outlined in Table 7.1, with grade 1 representing no need for treatment, to grade 5 representing a very great need for treatment.

These categories reflect need for treatment and thus health gain. When allocating a patient to a category the single worst feature of the malocclusion is chosen. For example, a class II division 1 incisor relationship with an overjet of greater than 9 mm is IOTN grade 5, that is, in very great need of treatment. As discussed previously, such a patient is at a greatly increased risk of incisal trauma, is more likely to suffer periodontal problems resulting from gingival dehydration and an increased overbite, and may well suffer from teasing, low expectations, and a low self-esteem.

Estimating the psychological impact of a malocclusion is where the second part of the index, the aesthetic component, is of use. However, the assessment is very subjective, especially for certain malocclusions. The ten pictures of malocclusion making up the aesthetic component are either class I or class II incisor relationships and it is therefore of limited use with other malocclusions, for example where the patient has a class III incisor relationship. Using the ten photographs of the aesthetic component (Fig. 7.2) the need for treatment is assessed as follows:

1 or 2 – no need for treatment

3 or 4 – slight need

5, 6, or 7 – moderate or borderline need

8, 9, or 10 – definite need for treatment.

Of the two parts of the IOTN, it is the dental health component that is in most frequent use.

It should be remembered that many of the presenting malocclusions are developmental dentofacial deformities, and not the result of self-neglect or abuse by the patient. Following diagnosis and

Table 7.1   Index of orthodontic treatment need, dental health component: for use on patients (reproduced with kind permission of the authors and the *European Journal of Orthodontics*)

Grade 5 – Very great need	Defects of cleft lip and/or palate Increased overjet greater than 9 mm Reverse overjet greater than 3.5 mm with reported masticatory or speech difficulties Impeded eruption of teeth (with the exception of third molars) due to crowding, displacement, the presence of supernumerary teeth, retained deciduous teeth, and any other pathological cause Extensive hypodontia with restorative implications (more than one tooth missing in any quadrant) requiring pre-restorative orthodontics
Grade 4 – Great need	Increased overjet greater than 6 mm but less than or equal to 9 mm Reverse overjet greater than 3.5 mm with no reported masticatory or speech difficulties Reverse overjet greater than 1 mm but less than or equal to 3.5 mm with reported masticatory or speech difficulties Anterior or posterior crossbites with greater than 2 mm displacement between retruded contact position and intercuspal position. Posterior lingual crossbites with no occlusal contact in one or both buccal segments Severe displacement of teeth greater than 4 mm Extreme lateral or anterior open bite greater than 4 mm Increased and complete overbite causing notable indentations on the palate or labial gingivae Patient referred by colleague for collaborative care (e.g. periodontal, restorative, or TMJ considerations) Less extensive hypodontia requiring pre-restorative orthodontics or orthodontic space closure to obviate the need for a prosthesis (not more than one tooth missing in any quadrant)
Grade 3 – Moderate need	Increased overjet greater than 3.5 mm but less than or equal to 6 mm with incompetent lips at rest

Table 7.1 *continued*

	Reverse overjet greater than 1 mm but less than or equal to 3.5 mm
	Increased and complete overbite with gingival contact but without indentations or signs of trauma
	Anterior or posterior crossbite with less than or equal to 2 mm but greater than 1 mm displacement between retruded contact position and intercuspal position
	Moderate lateral or anterior open bite greater than 2 mm but less than or equal to 4 mm
	Moderate displacement of teeth greater than 2 mm but less than or equal to 4 mm
Grade 2 – Little need	Increased overjet greater than 3.5 mm but less than or equal to 6 mm with lips competent at rest
	Reverse overjet greater than 0 mm but less than or equal to 1 mm
	Increased overbite greater than 3.5 mm with no gingival contact
	Anterior or posterior crossbite with less than or equal to 1 mm displacement between retruded contact position and intercuspal position
	Small lateral or anterior open bites greater than 1 mm but less than or equal to 2 mm
	Pre-normal or post-normal occlusions with no other anomalies
	Mild displacement of teeth greater than 1 mm but less than or equal to 2 mm
Grade 1 – No need	Other variations in occlusion including displacement less than or equal to 1 mm

treatment planning it is becoming increasingly common to allocate the patient to a treatment need category using the IOTN and thus determine whether treatment can be offered to them within a publicly funded health service. However, the determination of health gain is sometimes difficult, especially in the estimation of the psychosocial impact of malocclusion. Discretion is therefore required when setting priorities following the use of any index of treatment need.

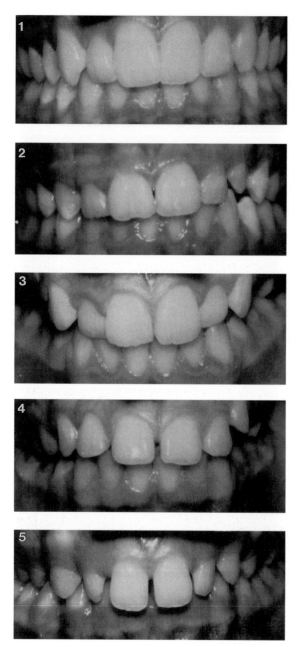

Fig. 7.2 The aesthetic component of the index of treatment need (IOTN).

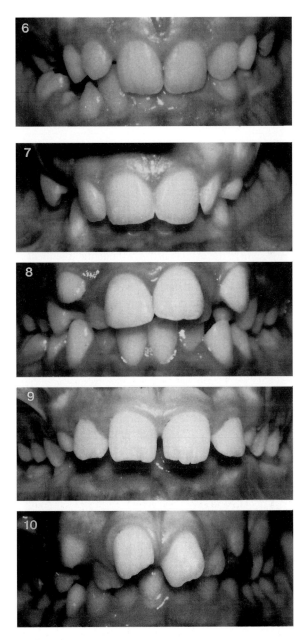

Fig. 7.2   *continued*

Summary of health considerations

Important health considerations are listed below.

1. Dental caries:
   (a) past
   (b) present
   (c) caries prevention.
2. Periodontal disease: consider the patient's age and assess using the CPITN probe.
3. Prevention of traumatic injury: this is related closely to the size of the overjet.
4. Psychosocial well-being.
5. Index of treatment need (IOTN): subdivided into the dental health and aesthetic components, it can be used as an aid when setting priorities where the availability of orthodontic treatment is limited.

Objectives

1. List the health considerations of importance in planning orthodontic treatment
2. List the basic categories of IOTN and the essential features of each grade

---

REFERENCES

1. Mirabella, A. D. and Årtun, J. (1995). Prevalence and severity of apical root resorption of maxillary anterior teeth in adult orthodontic patients. *European Journal of Orthodontics*, **17**, 93–9.
2. Kidd, E. A. M. and Joyston-Bechal, S. (1994). Update on fissure sealants. *Dental Update*, **21**, 323–6.
3. Kidd, E. A. M., Ricketts, D. N. J., and Pitts, N. B. (1993). Occlusal caries diagnosis: changing challenge for clinicians and epidemiologists. *Journal of Dentistry*, **21**, 323–31.
4. Sawle, R. F. and Andlaw, R. J. (1988). Has occlusal caries become more difficult to diagnose? *British Dental Journal*, **164**, 209–11.
5. Newbrun, E. (1989) *Cariology*, (3rd edn). Quintessence Books, Chicago.
6. Addy, M., Griffiths, G. S., Dummer, P. M. H., Kingdon, A., Hicks, R., Hunter, M., *et al.* (1988). The association between tooth irregularity

and plaque accumulation, gingivitis and caries in 11–12 year old children. *European Journal of Orthodontics*, **10**, 76–83.

7. Holloway, P. J. and Teagle, F. (1976). The relationship between oral cleanliness and caries increment. *Journal of Dental Research*, **55**, D106–No1.

8. Beal, J. F., James, P. M. C., Bradnock, G., and Anderson, R. J. (1979). The relationship between dental cleanliness, dental caries incidence and gingival health. A longitudinal study. *British Dental Journal*, **146**, 111–4.

9. WHO (1978). *Epidemiology, etiology and prevention of periodontal diseases*. Technical report series 621. World Health Organization, Geneva.

10. Löe, H. and Silness, J. (1963). Periodontal disease in pregnancy I. Prevalence and severity. *Acta Odontologica Scandinavica*, **21**, 533–51.

11. Löe, H. (1967). The gingival index, the plaque index and the retention index systems. *Journal of Periodontology*, **38** (Suppl.) 610–16.

12. Zachrisson, S. and Zachrisson, B. U. (1972). Gingival condition associated with orthodontic treatment. *Angle Orthodontist*, **42**, 26–34.

13. Lennon, M. A. and Davies, R. M. (1974). Prevalence and distribution of alveolar bone loss in a population of 15 year old schoolchildren. *Journal of Clinical Periodontology*, **1**, 175–82.

14. Zachrisson, B. U. and Alnæs, L. (1974). Periodontal condition in orthodontically treated and untreated individuals. II: alveolar bone loss; radiographic findings. *Angle Orthodontist*, **44**, 48–55.

15. Emslie, R. D., Massler, M., and Zwerner, J. D. (1952). Mouth breathing 1: Aetiology and effects. *Journal of the American Dental Association*, **44**, 506–21.

16. Palmer, R. M. and Floyd, P. D. (1995). Periodontology: a clinical approach. 1 Periodontal examination and screening. *British Dental Journal*, **178**, 185–9.

17. British Society of Periodontology (1994). *Periodontology in general dental practice in the United Kingdom*. A first policy statement. BSP,

18. Zachrisson, B. U. (1977). Clinical experience with direct-bonded orthodontic retainers. *American Journal of Orthodontics*, **71**, 440–8.

19. Eismann, D. and Prusas, R. (1990). Periodontal findings before and after orthodontic therapy in cases of incisor cross-bite. *European Journal of Orthodontics*, **12**, 281–3.

20. Ellis, R. G. (1960). *The classification and treatment of injuries to the teeth of children*, (4th edn). Year Book, Chicago.

21. Gutz, D. P. (1971). Fractured permanent incisors in a population. *Journal of Dentistry for Children*, **38**, 94–121.

22. Todd, J. E. and Dodd, T. (1985). *Children's dental health in the United Kingdom 1983*. Her Majesty's Stationery Office, London.

23. Hallett, G. E. M. (1953). Problems of common interest to the paedodontist and orthodontist with special reference to traumatised incisor cases. *Transactions of the European Orthodontic Society*, 266–77.

24. Eichenbaum, I. W. (1963). A correlation of traumatised anterior teeth to occlusion. *Journal of Dentistry for Children*, **30**, 229–36.
25. McEwen, J. D. and McHugh, W. D. (1969). Predisposing factors associated with fractured incisor teeth. *Transactions of the European Orthodontic Society*, 343–51.
26. Burden, D. (1995). An investigation of the association between overjet size, lip coverage, and traumatic injury to maxillary incisors. *European Journal of Orthodontics*, **17**, 513–17.
27. Shaw, W. C., Meek, S. C., and Jones D. S. (1980). Nicknames, teasing, harassment and salience of dental features among school children. *British Journal of Orthodontics*, **7**, 75–80.
28. Helm, S., Kreiborg, S., and Solow, B. (1985). Psychosocial implications of malocclusion. A 15 year follow up study in 30 year old Danes. *American Journal of Orthodontics*, **87**, 110–18.
29. Jenny, J. (1977). A social perspective on need and demand for orthodontic treatment. *International Dental Journal*, **25**, 248–56.
30. McGreggor, F. C. (1970). Social and psychological implications of dentofacial disfigurement. *Angle Orthodontist*, **40**, 231–3.
31. Byrne, D., London, O., and Reeves K. (1968). The effects of physical attractiveness, sex and attitude similarity on interpersonal attraction. *Journal of Personality*, **36**, 259–71.
32. Kleck, R. E. and Rubenstein, C. (1975). Physical attractiveness, perceived attitude similarity and interpersonal attraction in an opposite sex encounter. *Journal of Personal and Social Psychology*, **31**, 107–14.
33. Shaw, W. C. (1981). The influence of children's dentofacial appearance on their social attractiveness as judged by peers and lay adults. *American Journal of Orthodontics*, **79**, 399–415.
34. Kerosuo, H., Hausen, H., Laine, T., and Shaw W. C. (1995). The influence of incisal malocclusion on the social attractiveness of young adults in Finland. *European Journal of Orthodontics*, **17**, 505–12.
35. Clifford, M. M. (1975). Physical attractiveness and academic performance. *Child Studies Journal*, **5**, 201–9.
36. Brook, P. H. and Shaw, W. C. (1989). The development of an index of orthodontic treatment priority. *European Journal of Orthodontics*, **11**, 309–20.

8

Orthodontic records and diagnostic tests

A number of different types of records and diagnostic tests are required for orthodontic practice, each of which serves different purposes. These include.

(1) a written record of diagnosis, treatment planning, and treatment progress;

(2) orthodontic study models;

(3) radiographs; and

(4) photographs.

Other special investigations or diagnostic tests may also be performed. For example, teeth which have been previously traumatized should be tested for pulpal vitality and the results recorded.

Once records have been obtained they are used

(1) to aid initial diagnosis and treatment planning;

(2) for monitoring facial growth;

(3) for monitoring occlusal development;

(4) for monitoring treatment changes;

(5) for monitoring post-treatment changes;

(6) as a medico-legal requirement.

The various records and their functions will be discussed in turn.

8.1 WRITTEN RECORD OR CASE NOTES

The written record is an important legal record of the initial diagnosis, treatment planning, and the treatment progress of a case. For this reason, records should be thorough and yet concise. At no time should inappropriate comments be written in the notes about either the patient, their parents, or the treatment, as they may form part of the evidence available in court in cases of litigation.

The name of the patient, their address, and telephone number should obviously be recorded. During the initial diagnosis, the use of a pro forma (see Appendix 1) as the written record will ensure that no aspect of the examination of the patient is overlooked. Once the diagnosis and treatment plan have been determined they should be recorded clearly in the case notes. The treatment plan should follow a logical sequence, thereby making it relatively straightforward to monitor treatment progressing at any time. This is particularly important if the patient is to be transferred to another practitioner during the course of treatment. It is well established that a change of operator can prolong the duration of treatment. A clear record of the treatment plan and its progress can help to minimize this disruption as much as possible. At each appointment the clinical procedures performed should be recorded, along with the anticipated treatment procedure for the following appointment. This not only saves the clinician time, but enables the dental nurse to prepare the appropriate instruments and materials at the beginning of the next appointment, making for more efficient use of chair-side time.

8.2 ORTHODONTIC STUDY MODELS

Alginate impressions taken for orthodontic study models should be fully extended into the buccal sulcus using suitable impression trays. In this way the teeth and supporting alveolus will readily be visible on the subsequent plaster model. Using a wax wafer the position of the teeth in centric occlusion is also recorded so that the models can be hand articulated in the laboratory and Angle's trimmed. Such trimming enables the static occlusal relationships of the teeth to be studied by placing the models together on the bench at a number of different angles (Fig. 8.1).

Study models aid diagnosis in the following ways:

1. They enable occlusal relationships to be observed, which might not otherwise be visible. For example, where the overbite is

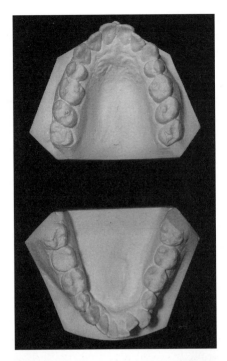

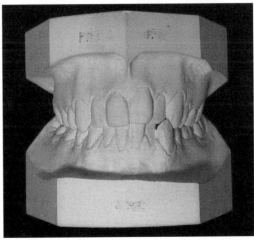

Fig. 8.1 This shows a set of study models correctly based and Angle's trimmed. They should be in maximum intercuspation if the distal edges of the models are coincident.

increased, the point of contact of the lower incisor edges with the opposing arch cannot be determined clinically and yet can easily be seen on the models.

2. An accurate space analysis can be performed using models, calipers, a millimetre rule, and a piece of soft wire. The wire is used to determine arch perimeter and the calipers are used in combination with the ruler to measure the mesiodistal widths of each of the teeth.

3. Models can be useful to both clinician and patient by demonstrating the effects of space closure, whether due to the developmental absence or planned extraction of teeth. Where teeth are developmentally absent the resulting space may either be closed or relocated within the arch. The effect of each treatment can be visualized by cutting the teeth off the models, moving them to the planned position and reattaching them with wax. This is known as a Kesling set-up (Fig. 8.2). Another instance where a Kesling set-up is recommended is in cases where a single lower incisor extraction is being planned. For example, in a case with lower incisor crowding, a class I incisor and molar relationship, and where the upper arch is well aligned, consideration might be given to a single lower incisor extraction. It will be important that this extraction provides sufficient space to align the remaining lower incisors and yet there is no residual space following treat-

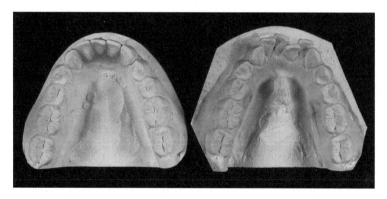

Fig. 8.2   A lower model before and after a Kesling set-up used to establish the feasibility of orthodontic treatment by removing a lower incisor.

ment. If any space should remain, then attempts to close it will lead to

(a) an increased overjet as the lower incisors are retroclined, or

(b) crowding in the upper incisor region as a result of the lower buccal segment teeth moving mesially into the residual space and cuspal interdigitation causing the upper buccal segment teeth also to move mesially.

Once orthodontic treatment has commenced, study models of the starting malocclusion are used to assess the progress of planned treatment changes. For example, they can be used to monitor changes in molar relationship during the distal movement of upper molars with a removable appliance and headgear. However, as well as being used to monitor changes in the occlusion, they are also useful as a reference to identify unwanted tooth movements. It is known that intercanine and intermolar widths within the same arch should remain constant throughout treatment in order to minimize relapse (see Chapter 9). Each time a new arch wire is placed during fixed appliance therapy, especially if the wires are preformed and used directly as supplied by the manufacturer, the intercanine and intermolar widths may be altered inadvertently. By referring back to the original study models, the arch wire can be adjusted prior to fitting in order to prevent any such unwanted expansion or contraction of the arch.

On completion of treatment, study models should be obtained as a record of the final result. Not only is such a record required for medico-legal purposes, but the pre and post-treatment models can be used to determine the PAR score (see Chapter 2) and thereby aid audit and quality control. The final models are subsequently used to monitor post-treatment changes in the occlusion.

In the same way that final models are taken at completion of treatment, in some cases models are taken but no treatment is undertaken at all. However, they can then be used to monitor changes with time, either to reassure the patient that development of the occlusion is continuing satisfactorily and that no active intervention is required, or to assist the patient in the decision making processes of whether to accept or reject orthodontic treatment.

8.3 RADIOGRAPHS

During diagnosis, radiographs are used to determine the following with regard to the teeth and supporting alveolus:

(1) presence

(2) position

(3) pathology.

In addition, the developmental stage of the teeth can also be determined.

Due to the unwanted side-effects of exposure to X-rays, the number of radiographs taken for any patient should be kept to a minimum, and only obtained when clinically necessary. Many radiographs are available to supplement the clinical examination and it is not the purpose of this text to repeat information already well documented elsewhere on radiography.[1] This chapter will concentrate on the views used most frequently by orthodontists. The three radiographs most commonly used during orthodontic diagnosis are a dental panoramic tomogram (DPT), an upper standard maxillary occlusal radiograph, and a lateral skull radiograph.

8.3.1 Dental panoramic tomogram (DPT)

This is also commonly referred to as an OPG or OPT. This rotational view (Fig. 8.3) utilizes the technique of tomography, whereby only a slice or section of the structure is viewed by coordinating the movement of the X-ray tube with the film in such a way as to mimic the horseshoe shape of the mandible. The DPT is notoriously poorly focused in the anterior maxillary region and for this reason its use is often supplemented with another view, namely the upper standard maxillary occlusal view. A major fault of the tomographic technique is the poor level of interpretation which is often applied to the image. They are not ideal views but can provide a considerable amount of information to the clinician. Typically they should be viewed and interpreted as follows.

1. A well-illuminated screen is essential for viewing, preferably with all ambient lighting eliminated except that passing through the radiograph.

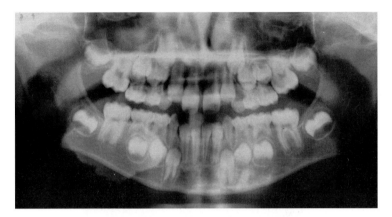

Fig. 8.3   A dental panoramic tomogram (DPT) used as a general overview of the occlusion. A point worthy of note in this case is the resorption on the mesial aspect of the maxillary deciduous canines reflecting a degree of crowding.

2. A standardized examination technique should be used, for example, starting posteriorly on the maxillary right, following around the arch to the left posterior maxilla and then repeating the process in the mandible. Bone density and alveolar bone levels can be examined first. The individual teeth are then studied. It is important to count the teeth, both erupted and unerupted, and to examine the crowns and roots in a systematic manner. As with many aspects of orthodontic diagnosis and treatment planning, it is important to look for symmetry in the structures.

3. Any abnormal anatomy seen from the rotational radiograph should be re-examined clinically and, where necessary, an accurate and clearly defined intra-oral radiograph taken. Interpretation of these latter radiographs is often helped not only by good illumination but also by a hand-held magnifying glass.

An alternative radiograph to the DPT, but one which serves the same purpose, is the bimolar view. This comprises two oblique lateral mandibular radiographs taken on one or two films (Fig. 8.4). Although usually lacking detail anterior to the canines, it can be taken with a less sophisticated and hence cheaper X-ray machine than is necessary for the DPT. The bimolar view can provide an exceptionally good view of the buccal segment teeth.

156

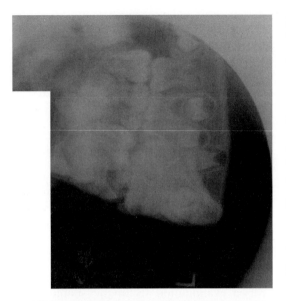

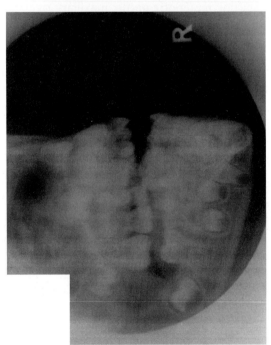

Fig. 8.4 A pair of oblique lateral mandibular views which can often be combined on one film. Again they offer an overview of the developing dentition.

However, obtaining a good radiograph does require more skill on the part of the operator than when using a DPT machine.

8.3.2 Upper standard maxillary occlusal radiograph

Also known as a nasal occlusal radiograph (Fig. 8.5), this is used to supplement the DPT which can suffer some loss of detail in the midline, a site where supernumerary teeth are frequently found.

8.3.3 Lateral skull radiograph

This radiograph (Fig. 8.6) is not taken routinely in the diagnosis of orthodontic cases but is usually obtained where there is a sagittal or vertical skeletal discrepancy. How such radiographs are interpreted is discussed later in section 8.6.

8.3.4 Other views

Where necessary, other views which may be obtained include bitewing radiographs, periapical radiographs, parallax views, the

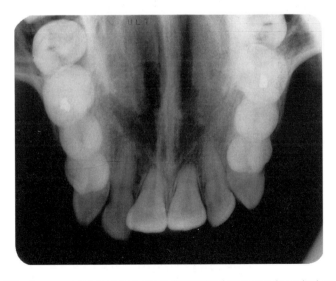

Fig. 8.5 An upper standard occlusal radiograph taken to see the apical area of the upper incisors in detail.

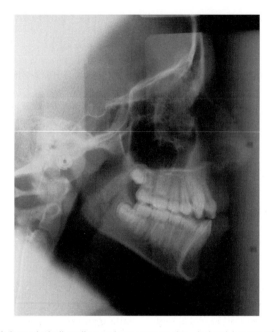

Fig. 8.6 A lateral skull radiograph to assess the skeletal bases of the facial skeleton. Notice the enhancement of the soft tissues by the presence of a wedge of aluminum.

postero-anterior skull radiograph, and vertex and mandibular occlusal radiographs.

Bitewing radiographs

These are used to help diagnose caries and, less often, to assess alveolar bone height.

Periapical radiographs

Following examination of the DPT it may be necessary to obtain a periapical radiograph in order to assess more accurately alveolar bone levels, root morphology, or other pathology. If a long cone periapical radiograph is taken in combination with a film holder, it can be used as a reference against which to measure any subsequent changes in root length, or alveolar bone levels during orthodontic treatment.

Parallax views

Such views are a combination of two radiographs taken at different angles. Using the principle of parallax, the position of an unerupted tooth relative to the adjacent, erupted teeth, can be determined. This principle is commonly used in the location of unerupted maxillary canines. The combination of views that can be used include the following:

1. Two periapical radiographs. In the location of a maxillary canine, the X-ray tube is moved horizontally around the arch by 10–20° between taking the two periapical radiographs. This is known as horizontal parallax (Fig. 8.7).

2. An upper standard occlusal and a periapical radiograph (Fig. 8.8). The principle is the same as with two periapical radiographs, with the upper standard occlusal assuming the role of one of the periapical radiographs.

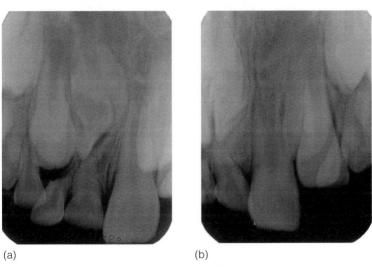

(a)   (b)

Fig. 8.7 A pair of periapical radiographs taken for assessment of a structure by parallax. In (a) the tip of the tuberculate shaped supernumerary tooth is lying close to the distal aspect of the upper right deciduous A. The contact point is clear between the left central incisor crown and the right deciduous tooth. In (b) the contact point is clear between the left central and lateral/supernumerary tooth. The tip of the tuberculate has moved with the X-ray tube, and is lying more to the middle of the upper right deciduous central incisor. Thus the tip must be palatal to this tooth.

3. An upper standard maxillary occlusal and a DPT (Fig. 8.9). In this case, instead of horizontal parallax, vertical parallax is used. This is possible because the DPT is taken with the X-ray beam at approximately 8° upwards to the occlusal plane whilst the upper standard maxillary occlusal is taken with the X-ray beam at approximately 70° to the occlusal plane.

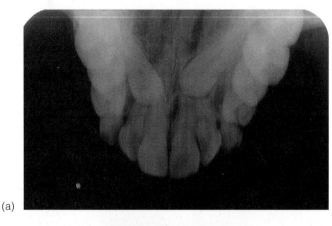

(a)

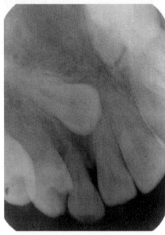

(b)

Fig. 8.8 A parallax pair of a standard occlusal and a periapical radiograph. In (a) the crown of the right maxillary canine is clearly overlying the apex of the upper right central incisor. Taking a new radiograph centred to the patient's right (b) shows the crown of the canine to be clear of the central. Thus the crown is palatal to the incisor root.

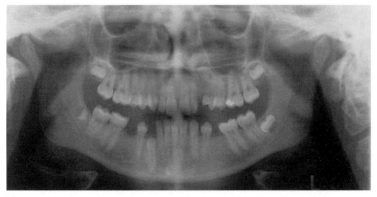

(a)

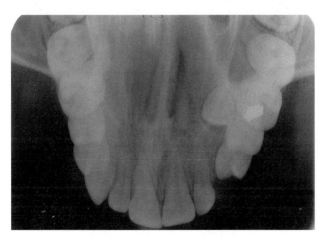

(b)

Fig. 8.9 An upper standard occlusal and a DPT utilizing vertical parallax. In the DPT view the tube is angled essentially parallel to the floor and the crown of the right maxillary canine is seen to be distant to the incisor apices. In the standard occlusal the tube moves upwards and the crown is seen to move towards the incisor apices. This is in the opposite direction to the X-ray tube and so the canine crown is buccal to the incisor apices.

In the principle of parallax, the object closest to the film moves in the same direction as the X-ray tube. Many acronyms exist and it is only required that each person remembers the one that they can readily recollect. Such *aides-mémoire* include 'buccal/away, palatal/same', referring to the fact that if the crown of an unerupted tooth moves in the same direction as the X-ray tube it is palatal and *vice versa*. This is outlined in Figs 8.7–8.9.

Postero-anterior skull radiograph

This is rarely taken for the purposes of orthodontic diagnosis. In combination with a lateral skull radiograph, the two views, which are perpendicular to each other, can be used to locate unerupted teeth, such as the maxillary canine. However, the views discussed previously, especially the combination of the upper standard occlusal and the DPT are more commonly used, since they are taken routinely for orthodontic diagnosis in any case. The postero-anterior skull view is occasionally used to assess cases in which there is a marked mandibular asymmetry and where surgery is being contemplated.

Vertex occlusal radiograph

This infrequently taken view can be helpful in determining whether an unerupted canine is palatally or buccally positioned relative to the incisor teeth. However, it has a number of disadvantages, including being difficult to take, limited in the amount of information it provides, as well as involving a relatively high dose of radiation to the patient.

Mandibular occlusal radiograph

This view is occasionally used for the localization of unerupted teeth such as ectopic mandibular canines.

8.4 PHOTOGRAPHS

Colour photographs can be an extremely valid record, especially for medico-legal purposes as a record of the pre and post-treatment condition of the enamel surfaces of the teeth. Photographs can be taken with the teeth in occlusion, anteriorly, as well as right and left lateral views. Mirrors can be used to obtain upper and lower occlusal views of the arches. Defects on the enamel surfaces of particular teeth can be taken as separate photographs at a higher magnification. As well as intra-oral views, extra-oral photographs can also be obtained. These are usually full face and profile as well as a three-quarter view, which is the lateral view most often seen by the patient of their own face and of others in social contact.

Scaled intra-oral photographs can be used in a similar way to study models, both before and after treatment. Extra-oral photographs are more limited, due to the reproducibility of facial expression. Certainly intra-oral photographs, if they were to be accepted as a substitute for study models, would overcome the storage problems of the latter. There is currently a legal requirement for study models to be retained many years after completion of treatment. With the advent of digital photography and the ability to store many such images on computer, it may only be a question of time before such records replace study models in orthodontic practise, despite the legal considerations that exist at present.

8.5 OTHER DIAGNOSTIC TESTS OR SPECIAL INVESTIGATIONS

Other less frequently used tests and records used in orthodontic diagnosis include vitality testing, transillumination, hand-wrist radiographs, and articulation/occlusal registration.

8.5.1 Vitality testing

Teeth may be vitality tested with either chloroethane (ethyl chloride) or an electric pulp tester. A more recent advance includes laser Doppler flowmetry. This can be performed whenever tooth vitality is in question and the results carefully recorded in the case notes.

8.5.2 Transillumination

This can be performed when a tooth has previously suffered trauma, in order to detect the presence of any enamel infraction lines. This might be especially appropriate when ceramic, fixed appliance brackets are to be used on such teeth. It can be very difficult to remove these brackets at completion of treatment without damaging normal enamel, let alone previously damaged enamel.

8.5.3 Hand–wrist radiographs

These radiographs are used in an attempt to identify ossification of the phalanxes and in so doing assist in the assessment of the pubertal growth spurt. Many reviews of this type of radiographic image have been written[2,3] and while ossification dates are of value in a limited numbers of cases, for the vast majority of patients the ossification events are identified too late to be of use in orthodontic treatment.

8.5.4 Articulation/occlusal registration

The role of articulated models in orthodontic diagnosis, other than Angle's trimmed study models, has been discussed in Chapter 6. The standard records are hand articulated Angle's trimmed study models. The purpose of such trimming is to enable the static occlusion to be observed from several different angles.

Further tests and records, such as those to assess periodontal disease and tooth mobility, are discussed in Chapter 5.

8.6 CEPHALOMETRICS

Lateral skull radiographs are used as the basis of the science of cephalometrics in which the angulation of dental structures, as well as the positions of the underlying skeletal bases with respect to the remainder of the facial skeleton, are measured. Points or landmarks are identified on the radiograph from which angular and, less often, linear measurements are made. This is completed, either by tracing the radiograph using a pencil, paper, and a protractor, or by digitizing the radiograph using a digitizer linked to a personal computer and analysed with the appropriate software. The cephalometric analysis has four main purposes, namely diagnosis, prediction, prescription, and research. These will each be dealt with in turn.

8.6.1 Diagnosis

There is no substitute for a thorough clinical assessment of a patient in the determination of an orthodontic diagnosis. The lateral skull radiograph and subsequent cephalometric analysis should always be considered an adjunct to this assessment, not a substitute. While some commercial organizations claim to be able to plan treatment on the basis of study models and lateral skull radiographs alone, the treatment plans provided are less than satisfactory. As an adjunctive tool, the lateral skull radiograph will help to determine how the various aetiological agents might be interacting to produce the malocclusion in question.

8.6.2 Prediction

In planning certain types of orthodontic treatment it is important to be able to predict either the beginning or the end of a period of growth, or whether the patient is likely to grow in a certain manner. For example, if functional appliances are to be used to correct a class II skeletal relationship, these are most effective if they are worn during the pubertal growth spurt, when facial growth is rapid. Orthognathic surgery, on the other hand, usually cannot be performed until facial growth has ceased. As well as predicting these two events it is useful to be able to predict the manner or direction of growth. For instance, is the patient going to show an anterior or posterior growth rotation? Whereas lateral skull radiographs are of limited use in the prediction of the start of the pubertal growth spurt, they can be used to determine when facial growth has all but ceased. Serial radiographs, taken over a number of years and compared with each other, can help determine when an event has passed, but not when an event is about to take place. Similarly, in determining the manner or direction of growth, serial radiographs and analyses can only determine that a type of growth has occurred. Indications that a type of growth is to occur, or as is more likely, is already occurring, can be gleaned from the initial radiograph and analysis. Therefore, a patient with an increased anterior lower facial height, an increased Frankfort–mandibular planes angle or maxillary–mandibular planes angle, and who demonstrates a pronounced gonial notch on the lower border of the mandible is likely to have a posterior mandibular growth rotation, which will continue until facial growth is complete (see Fig. 4.9).

8.6.3 Prescription

The assessment of skeletal pattern and inclination of the labial segment teeth will assist in treatment prescription. It will help determine whether an overjet can be treated by simply tipping the upper labial segment teeth with a removable appliance or whether bodily movement using fixed appliances is necessary. It will also help determine whether functional appliances or perhaps orthognathic surgery is required to correct an underlying skeletal discrepancy. Although the lateral skull radiograph and cephalometric analysis will assist in the prescription of treatment it should not be used as the only means of prescription, or as a substitute for a thorough and systematic clinical examination. For instance, in a class II division 1 incisor relationship on a class II skeletal base, the cephalometric analysis might suggest that an upper removable appliance can be used to reduce the overjet and create a class I incisor relationship (Fig. 8.10). In this case the upper incisors are proclined at the start of treatment. What the radiograph and cephalometric analysis cannot provide is information on crowding or spacing within the arches, the angulation of, for example, the upper canines, or the presence of multiple tooth rotations, all of which might require fixed appliances for correction.

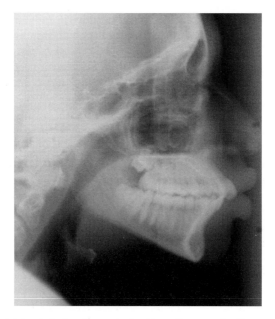

Fig. 8.10 A lateral skull radiograph of a bimaxillary proclination case showing good contrast of the soft tissues including that in the pharyngeal area.

However, a word of caution should be emphasized at this point. It is totally inappropriate to prescribe a treatment plan on the basis of the cephalometrics alone and both authors would strongly advise clinicians to avoid this. Patients should not be treated to population 'norms' but these figures should be used as a guide in identifying the aetiology of a malocclusion. This is particularly necessary not only in considering the range of normal variation but also when examining patients from differing ethnic backgrounds for whom cephalometric norms do not apply. Each patient should be assessed clinically and the cephalometric analysis used to support or refute the clinical findings. On no account should a diagnosis and treatment plan be formulated on the basis of a cephalometric analysis alone.

In addition to aiding prescription at the beginning of orthodontic treatment, a lateral skull radiograph and cephalometric analysis are sometimes obtained mid-treatment. This may be necessary to monitor treatment progress and help determine whether any other appliances are required.

8.6.4 Research

Cephalometric analyses are many and varied and have been used to investigate both facial growth and the influence orthodontic treatment might have on the process. Research using lateral skull radiographs began in the early 1930s[4] and subsequent longitudinal growth studies[5,6] have helped not only in the understanding of facial growth, but have enabled average values for different facial dimensions to be established, against which a patient can be compared. Although average values are available, treatment should never be planned on the basis of making the patient fit these values.

It is not essential to obtain a lateral skull radiograph for each and every prospective orthodontic patient. The radiograph and any subsequent analysis is unlikely to be of great diagnostic benefit in cases where the anteroposterior or vertical skeletal relationships are normal, or only mildly incorrect, and where there is a class I incisor relationship. In other circumstances the lateral skull radiograph and associated cephalometric analysis form a useful diagnostic tool when used in conjunction with a full orthodontic clinical examination.

In order to carry out a cephalometric analysis a number of standards should be met in obtaining and subsequently studying the radiograph.

1. The radiograph should be taken in a standardized manner. The patient's head should be placed in a cephalostat and the mid-sagittal plane of the patient should be parallel with the plane of the film. The central X-ray beam should be perpendicular to this plane and passing through the ear rods used to orientate the patient within the cephalostat. The distances from the X-ray tube to the mid-sagittal plane of the patient, and from the latter to the film, are usually set at 2 m and less than 0.3 m respectively. Any variation in these distances will affect the magnification of the final image. Generally, magnification is restricted to be within 5–12 per cent. In order to enhance of the soft tissue profile image, an aluminium wedge is placed between the patient and the X-ray tube. In addition, a moving grid between the patient and film will improve picture quality by reducing the effect of X-ray scatter as the beam passes through the patient.

2. The final radiograph should be viewed on an X-ray viewer which is capable of providing an even light source.

3. The radiograph should be orientated on the viewer with the Frankfort plane horizontal. This is essential, as many of the cephalometric landmarks are defined as points on an arc of a circle. For example, point A (Fig. 8.11), which represents the anterior border of the maxilla (see list below), is defined as the innermost point on the concavity between the anterior nasal spine and the labial alveolar crest of the upper incisors. Tilting the radiograph so that the Frankfort plane is not horizontal will markedly affect the position of point A.

4. The radiograph should be viewed in a darkened room, eliminating any light from the X-ray viewer which is *not* passing through the radiograph.

5. It is possible to perform the analysis directly by digitizing the radiograph, using a digitizer linked to a computer. There are a number of computer programs available for this purpose. Alternatively, landmarks can be identified and traced using good quality tracing paper and a sharp 4H pencil. Measurements are then taken from the tracing using a ruler and a protractor.

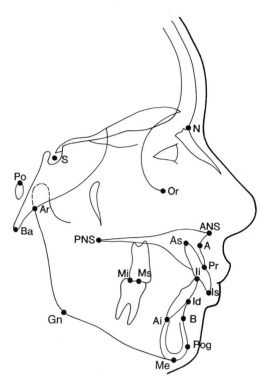

Fig. 8.11 A lateral skull tracing with some of the most commonly used points outlined (see text for details).

In this book only a basic analysis will be described and texts dedicated to cephalometric analyses should be consulted for a more detailed insight into this subject.[1] However, it is worth remembering that many analyses are available, indicating that cephalometry is an inexact science. As such it must not be used as a diagnostic tool in isolation from a thorough clinical examination.

A basic analysis is illustrated in Fig. 8.12. Angular measurements are commonly used in preference to linear measurements because the former are affected to a lesser extent by both the equipment used to obtain the radiograph and also by facial growth. The points of interest for the basic analysis and their definitions are as follows.

1. Orbitale (Or) – the most inferior anterior point on the border of the orbit. This can be a difficult landmark to locate.

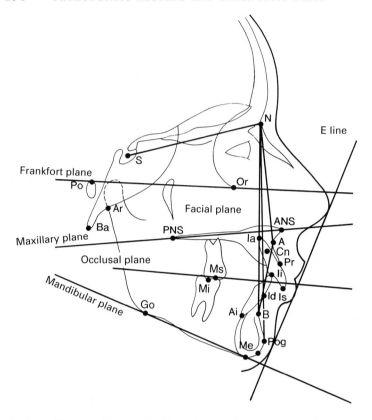

Fig. 8.12 The same figure as 8.11 but with the relevant planes outlined.

2. Porion (Po) – the superior border of the external auditory meatus. This can be a difficult landmark to locate.

3. Sella or point S – this is the middle of the sella turcica and is easily identified.

4. Nasion or point N – this is the innermost point on the concavity between the frontal and nasal bones. In a young individual where the fronto-nasal suture is still patent, nasion is the most anterior point on the suture.

5. point A – the innermost point on the concavity between the anterior nasal spine and the labial alveolar crest of the upper incisors. It serves as the anterior reference point of the maxilla

but is not situated on basal bone. Being on alveolar bone its position can change as a result of remodelling of the alveolus during tooth movement. This needs to be remembered when interpreting treatment changes on pre and post-treatment radiographs.

6. Pogonion (Pog) – the most anterior point on the bony chin.

7. point B – the innermost point on the concavity between the alveolar crest of the most prominent lower incisor and pogonion.

8. Menton (Me) – the most inferior point on the bony symphysis of the chin.

9. Gonion (Gn) – the most posterior inferior point at the angle of the mandible.

10. Anterior nasal spine ANS – this can be difficult to locate unless an aluminium wedge has been used to improve the soft tissue profile image, in which case ANS also becomes more readily visible.

11. Posterior nasal spine PNS – this can be difficult to locate, especially in the presence of unerupted upper third permanent molars. In this case the position of PNS is taken as the intersect of a line passing through the pterygomaxillary fissure perpendicular with a line passing through the middle of the palate and parallel with the floor of the nose.

12. Incisal edge of the most prominent upper central incisor (Is).

13. Apex of the most prominent upper central incisor (Ia).

14. Incisal edge of the most prominent lower central incisor (Ii).

15. Apex of the most prominent lower central incisor (Ai).

16. Centroid of the root of the most prominent incisor (Cn). The centroid is taken as the midpoint on the root between the root apex and the junction between the root and crown of the tooth.

17. Basion (Ba) – the most posterior inferior point on the basi-occiput.

18. Articulare (Ar) – the intersection of the posterior border of the neck of the mandibular condyle and the lower margin of the posterior cranial base.

19. Molar superioris (Ms) – the most concave aspect of the crown of the maxillary molar.

20. Molar inferioris (Mi) – the most concave aspect of the crown of the mandibular molar.

Other points are included but are of limited value to non-specialist analysis.

During the extra-oral examination of a patient the Frankfort plane is used as a substitute for the maxillary plane because, unlike the maxillary plane, it is easy to locate. When a lateral skull radiograph is obtained for analysis, the picture is taken with the patient's head in the free-postural position and with the Frankfort plane horizontal. It is therefore desirable to orientate the radiograph prior to analysis with the Frankfort plane horizontal. However, as discussed, the two points used to construct this plane are difficult to locate on a radiograph. If difficulty is experienced then the radiograph can be orientated using the maxillary plane, since not only can the maxillary plane be accurately located on the radiograph, but the two planes are closely correlated. Once the radiograph has been orientated, the following lines and angles are constructed.

1. The line S–N. This is used as the stable reference against which maxillary and mandibular prominence are recorded. It is used as such because the anterior cranial base with which it is associated will alter little after 6–7 years of age, when neural growth will have ceased along with fusion of the spheno-ethmoidal synchondrosis. Limitations of its use, however, include closure of the fronto-nasal suture and a subsequent redefinition of the point nasion. Nasion is also located at the junction of two bones which undergo surface remodelling, particularly during puberty in males.

2. Angle SNA. Normally this angle measures $82 \pm 3°$ and is a measure of maxillary prominence. It suffers from the inherent inaccuracies of the line S–N, identification of point A, and the fact that point A may move as a result of alveolar remodelling during treatment.

3. Angle SNB. Normally this angle measures $79 \pm 3°$. This suffers from the same inaccuracies as experienced in the determination of the angle SNA.

4. Angle ANB. This angle will give an indication of skeletal pattern as follows:

    (a) 2 – 4° is a class I skeletal pattern;
    (b) > 4° a class II skeletal pattern; and
    (c) < 2° a class III skeletal pattern.

    It should be noted that variations in the position of nasion can affect the angle ANB. If the angle SNA deviates markedly form the normal range, then the angle ANB should be interpreted with some caution. It is possible to correct for discrepancies in the angle SNA. Provided the angle SN to maxillary plane is within the range 8 ± 3° then the value of ANB can be adjusted to account for variations in the angle SNA. For every degree the angle SNA is greater than 82°, then 0.5° can be subtracted from the angle ANB, and *vice versa* for every degree the angle SNA is below 82°.

5. The maxillary plane is a line joining ANS and PNS.

6. The mandibular plane is a line joining menton to gonion.

7. The maxillary mandibular planes angle (MMA). This normally measures 27 ± 5°.

8. The inclination of the most prominent upper incisor to the maxillary plane (1MxP). The long axis of the most prominent upper incisor is constructed by joining the two points, upper incisor edge (Is) and upper incisor apex (Ia). The angle this line makes with the maxillary plane is then determined and usually measures 108 ± 5°.

9. The inclination of the most prominent lower incisor to the mandibular plane (1̄MnP). The long axis of the most prominent lower incisor is constructed by joining the two points, lower incisor edge (Ii) and lower incisor apex (Ai). The angle made with the mandibular plane is then determined and normally measures 92 ± 5°.

10. The interincisal angle. This is the angle between the long axis of the most prominent upper incisor and the most prominent lower incisor and is normally 133 ± 10°.

11. Lower incisor edge to upper root centroid distance. This normally measures 0 – 2 mm and serves as a useful tool not only in the explanation of overbite, but also in the tooth movements required to correct the incisor relationship.[7]

12.   Anterior lower face height (ALFH) as a percentage of overall face height. Using the maxillary plane, two perpendiculars are constructed, one to menton and one to nasion. These two distances added together constitute total face height, and the distance menton to maxillary plane is then calculated as a percentage of this total. Normally ALFH comprises 55 per cent of the total anterior face height.

This straightforward cephalometric analysis is useful in assessing anteroposterior and vertical skeletal relationships, as well as the relationship of the upper and lower incisors to their skeletal bases and to each other. In this way not only will it serve as an adjunct to the impression gained by the clinical examination, but will help in the planning of tooth movements, particularly in the labial segments.

8.7 BALLARD'S CONVERSION

This technique can assist in understanding the complex nature of craniofacial growth and the potential adaptation which occurs during life.[8] It requires the standard cephalometric tracing, followed by a 'normalization' of the upper and lower incisor inclinations. That is, the incisors are rotated about their centroid (see Glossary), one-third down from the root apex, to the ideal inclination. Once in the new positions the overjet is reassessed with the teeth in the non-compensatory positions. This gives a clearer indication of the severity of the underlying anteroposterior skeletal pattern and can assist treatment planning.

Summary of orthodontic records and diagnostic tests

Records required for orthodontic diagnosis and subsequent treatment include
(1)   written records of diagnosis, treatment planning, and treatment progress;
(2)   orthodontic study models;

Summary of orthodontic records and diagnostic tests
(continued)

(3) radiographs (the DPT, upper standard maxillary occlusal, and lateral skull are the most frequently used. Other views may be used for determining unerupted tooth position or when investigating caries and periodontal disease);

(4) photographs (particularly useful as a record of enamel condition).

These records serve the following purposes.

1. To aid initial diagnosis and treatment planning
2. For monitoring facial growth
3. For monitoring occlusal development
4. For monitoring treatment changes
5. For monitoring post-treatment changes
6. As a medico-legal requirement

Cephalometric analysis

This is performed on a lateral skull radiograph and the angular and linear measurements can be used in

- diagnosis
- prediction of growth
- prescription of treatment
- research into growth or treatment effects

Objectives

1. List possible special tests used in diagnosis
2. Identify and define the points commonly used in cephalometric analysis
3. Recall how to obtain a parallax pair of radiographs and interpret these

REFERENCES

1. Whaites, E. (1996). *Essentials of dental radiography and radiology*, (2nd edn). Churchill Livingstone, Edinburgh.

2. Houston, W. J. B. (1980). Relationships between skeletal maturity estimated from hand–wrist radiographs and the timing of the adolescent growth spurt. *European Journal of Orthodontics*, **2**, 81–93.
3. Sullivan, P. G. (1983). Prediction of the pubertal growth spurt by measurement of standing height. *European Journal of Orthodontics*, **5**, 189–97.
4. Broadbent, B. H. (1931). A new X-ray technique and its application to orthodontics. *Angle Orthodontist*, **1**, 45–66.
5. Broadbent, B. H. (1937). The face of the normal child: Bolton standards and technique. *Angle Orthodontist*, **7**, 183–233.
6. Björk, A. and Skieller, V. (1983). Normal and abnormal growth of the mandible. A synthesis of longitudinal cephalometric implant studies over a 25 year period. *European Journal of Orthodontics*, **5**, 1–46.
7. Houston, W. J. B. (1989). The incisor edge–centroid relationship and overbite depth. *European Journal of Orthodontics* **11**, 139–43.
8. Ballard, C. F. (1967). The morphological bases of prognosis determination and treatment planning. *British Society for the Study of Orthodontics*, 95–106.

SUGGESTED FURTHER READING

Athanasioic, A. E. (1995). *Orthodontic cephalometry* Mosby Wolfe, London.
Isaacson, K. G. and Jones M. L. (1994). *Orthodontic radiography*. British Orthodontic Society.

9

Evidence based practice

In both medicine and dentistry many of the available treatments in use by clinicians are based on personal training, clinical experience, the authoritative views of colleagues, or as a result of research findings. Such a varied background can lead to slow acceptance of new and effective treatment modalities by clinicians as a whole, and, equally, outdated and ineffective treatments may only slowly be discarded. The purpose of an evidence based approach to dentistry, involving clinical decision making based on known evidence, is to overcome such problems. Thus clinical problems are dealt with by gathering evidence, systematically evaluating it, and then acting upon it where appropriate rather than relying on, the anecdotal evidence of others. The evidenced based process should be ongoing with fresh evidence being evaluated as it becomes available. Published evidence can be ranked from just a single case report, up to the ideal of a systematic review of multiple, well-designed, randomized controlled clinical trials. The stated advantages of evidence based dentistry are[1]

(1) to improve the effective use of research evidence in clinical practice, where hopefully new and more effective treatments will be more readily introduced. Likewise, ineffective treatments will be rejected;

(2) to enable more effective use of resources;

(3) to rely on evidence rather than authority (i.e. views of others) in making clinical decisions, thereby helping to ensure more up to date practice;

(4) to enable a practitioner to monitor and subsequently develop their own clinical performance either through audit or by contributing to more formalized research.

There may, however, be difficulties with rigidly applying an evidenced based approach to clinical practice. It can be very time intensive for an individual clinician when solving clinical problems, and indeed it may stifle innovation if purchasing authorities insist on clinicians following rigid proven treatment regimens in all forms, be it in method or materials.

Within orthodontics, evidence based practice can be dealt with under a number of headings, including

(1) indications for orthodontic treatment;

(2) effectiveness of different treatment modalities;

(3) orthodontic materials;

(4) stability following orthodontic treatment; and

(5) iatrogenic damage as a result of orthodontic treatment.

Some of the scientific evidence related to health as an indication for orthodontic treatment has been discussed in Chapter 7, whilst the effectiveness of specific treatment modalities and orthodontic materials are beyond the scope of this book. The evidence base concerning stability following orthodontic treatment will be discussed further, as it is an important consideration in diagnosis and treatment planning.

9.1 LABIOLINGUAL POSITIONING OF THE LOWER INCISORS

The positioning of the lower incisors for long term stability in orthodontic treatment planning has been a controversial topic for many years. A great deal of work has been published, both anecdotal and more scientifically-based, which only seems to confirm the complex nature of the subject. Various clinicians have put their names to cephalometric analyses[2,3] devised to help in planning the post-treatment labiolingual position of the lower incisors. However, the problem with most of these analyses is that they aim to place the lower incisors into a position which will give a good aesthetic result, with little or no attention being paid to long term stability. A study on stability[4,5] using the angular measurement SNIi on lateral skull radiographs (Fig. 9.1) found that whether proclined or retroclined, lower incisors tended to return to their pretreatment position once all orthodontic appliances were removed. A subsequent review of the literature[6] recommended a cautious approach to labiolingual movement of the lower incisors in treatment planning, along the

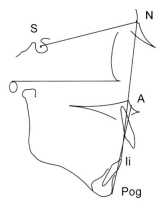

Fig. 9.1 A line drawing illustrating the angle SNIi (sella–nasion to the incisal edge of the lower central incisor) and the line A–Pog (the line joining point A to pogonion).

lines advocated.[4,5] However, it was still suggested that the relationship of the lower incisors to the A–Pog line[7] would be a useful guide in planning, producing both a stable and an aesthetically pleasing result. The stated aim was to place the lower incisor edges within 2 mm of the A–Pog line at the end of active orthodontic treatment. Advantages of using this line are said to be its proximity to the lower incisors compared with other cephalometric analyses and the ease with which it can be used at the chair-side. A retrospective analysis of treated cases up to 20 years out of retention[8] has once again shown that even this simple analysis is flawed. On the whole, the lower incisors have a tendency to return towards their pretreatment labiolingual position, irrespective of the relationship of the lower incisors to the A–Pog line. To complicate matters, the extent to which labiolingual relapse takes place is not dependent upon how far the lower incisors are moved from their pretreatment position. In other words, those cases in which the lower incisors are moved furthest labiolingually during treatment do not necessarily demonstrate the greatest degree of relapse.

It would seem that there are no currently available predictors of long term labiolingual lower incisor stability. The best advice would still seem to be to accept the current pretreatment labiolingual position as being the most likely stable position, although even then this is not an absolute guide to long term stability. The only real guarantee would be permanent retention, in one form or another. This might be with a bonded wire retainer, lingual to the lower incisors, or a removable retainer worn on a part time basis, both of which may have dental health implications for the teeth and their supporting structures.

Generally agreed exceptions to maintaining the initial labio-lingual position of the lower incisors in orthodontic treatment planning and subsequent treatment are listed below.

1. Retroclination of the lower incisors in class III incisor relationships where initially there was a reverse overjet and where there will be a positive overbite at the end of treatment capable of retaining the new incisor position. It should be noted that before treating such a case by lower incisor retroclination, other factors such as skeletal pattern and incisor inclination must also be considered (see Chapter 10).

2. Proclination may be permissible where there is trapping of the lower incisors in the palate in a class II division 1 incisor relationship, and where it is presumed that the lower incisors have been prevented from expressing their true, more anterior, labiolingual position (Fig. 9.2). This may also include some class II division 2 incisor relationships.

3. Proclination again may be permissible where there has been a history of a persistent digit sucking habit. The habit may have caused retroclination of the lower incisors and proclination of the upper incisors, which is perpetuated by an adaptive soft tissue behaviour on swallowing after cessation of the habit. Correction of the incisor position will hopefully lead to normal soft tissue behaviour, maintaining a stable correction of the incisors.

The problem with all these exceptions, and in particular with the second and third, is that there is still no way of predicting how much the labiolingual position of the lower incisors can be altered and yet a stable result achieved.

9.2 LOWER INCISOR ALIGNMENT

One of the major indications for undertaking orthodontic treatment is to obtain an aesthetic improvement; correcting tooth malalignment is one of the ways in which this is achieved. When considering

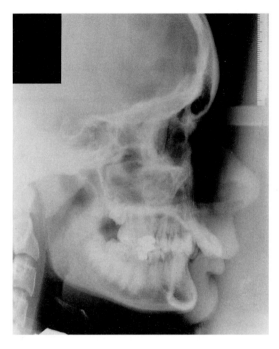

Fig. 9.2 Lower incisor trapping in this class II division 1 incisor relationship has prevented true expression of lower incisor position. In such cases proclination of the lower incisors may be acceptable and stable.

post-treatment stability of the lower incisors, alignment and labio-lingual position are two separate and important factors which do not necessarily go hand in hand. Investigations into the stability of the labiolingual position found a tendency of the lower incisors to move back towards their pretreatment labiolingual position when all appliances had been removed. However, this did not always lead to a simultaneous deterioration in the alignment of the teeth.[8] Post-treatment stability of dental arch alignment has been extensively studied at the University of Washington, Seattle, with cases treated using fixed appliances being evaluated at least 10 years post-retention. A disappointing finding is that more than 60 per cent of cases will demonstrate an unacceptable level of deterioration in lower incisor alignment post-retention.[9] This has subsequently been confirmed in other studies.[10,11]

In order to understand long term relapse it is necessary to consider the physiological changes that occur with age in untreated normal occlusions from the early permanent dentition through to early adulthood. Both arch length and intercanine width typically decrease with age, while changes in intermolar width are more variable. There is usually a slight increase in intermolar width in males with increasing age and a decrease in width in females. These changes, especially the decrease in arch length and intercanine width, are usually associated with the increase in lower incisor crowding seen in the late teenage years.[12] However, these normal physiological changes do not cease in the late teens, but continue for many years afterwards,[13] often beyond the age of 40 years, albeit at a reduced rate.[14] Both the reduction in arch length and late lower incisor crowding are related to facial growth. Generally the mandible is considered to grow in a downwards and forwards direction, but superimposed upon this, both the mandible and the maxilla may undergo growth rotations. These rotations have been demonstrated on serial lateral skull radiographs, using subperiosteal titanium implants as fixed reference markers,[15] and are due to differential growth in anterior and posterior face height.[16] The effect on the occlusion of continued facial growth and growth rotations is largely masked by dento-alveolar adaptation. However, it is precisely this adaptation which may lead to changes in the alignment of teeth, whilst still maintaining the overall occlusal contacts between the upper and lower arch teeth.

The degree to which the aforementioned changes will occur is very variable, and there are no predictors to enable the clinician to know which cases will deteriorate unacceptably with time. The only way of guaranteeing that teeth remain aligned after active orthodontic treatment is to retain the result, perhaps on a part time but indefinite basis. Cases which show the greatest tendency towards lower incisor stability are those which initially present with generalized spacing and where this spacing is closed during treatment.[17] In this instance there is approximately a 50 per cent chance of the lower incisors remaining acceptably aligned up to 10 years post-retention. It should be noted, however, that even in this type of case, almost 50 per cent of patients will still have unacceptable alignment of the lower incisors 10 years out of retention, presumably because the narrowing of the intercanine width and reduction in arch length seen in other patients still occurs. The

third permanent molars have also been suggested as possible con-
tributors to late lower incisor crowding and are discussed later.

9.3 CORRECTION OF INCISOR RELATIONSHIP

A frequent aim of orthodontic treatment is to produce or maintain
a class I incisor relationship. For class II and III incisor relationships this will entail either tipping or bodily movement of the upper
incisors, often preceded by an alteration of the overbite. Most of the
studies looking at the stability of correction of incisor relationships
have been retrospective, on previously treated class I and class II
division 1 incisor relationships, many years out of retention.
Treatment modalities have included fixed appliance therapy with
and without extractions[18-21] as well as functional appliance
therapy.[22] Generally, increases in overjet and overbite following
incisor correction have been found to be very small. Mean overjet
changes between 0.5 mm and 2 mm have been quoted, whilst
mean overbite changes have varied between 0.9 mm and 3 mm.
Criticisms of some studies are that too few cases are included and
the diversity of the initial malocclusions is often great. Therefore,
although the mean changes in overbite and overjet might be small
there is often a wide range of recorded values. The relationship
between initial overbite and overjet and the tendency to relapse is
not clear. Stability will depend on several factors including, in the
short term, skeletal pattern and lip competence. In the longer term
the factors affecting stability are discussed under labiolingual position and alignment of the lower incisors and are probably related to
continued facial growth. The incisor changes that are said to lead
to the relapse in overbite and overjet have been listed as

(1) proclination of the upper incisors

(2) occlusal movement of the upper incisors

(3) occlusal movement of the lower incisors

(4) retroclination of the lower incisors.

In the case of treated class II division 2 incisor relationships, statistically significant degrees of relapse of overbite and interincisal
angle towards their pretreatment values have been described in
cases five years out of all retaining appliances.[23] A major cause of

relapse in such cases is, once again, probably continued facial growth. As a result, retroclination of the upper and the lower incisors occurs, leading to an increase in the interincisal angle and consequently an increase in the overbite. Although quoted as statistically significant, the mean relapse, measured both in degrees and in millimetres for both the interincisal angle and the overbite is small, and probably not clinically significant.[23] With the many variables involved in the maintenance of a corrected class I and class II incisor relationship, including orthodontic relapse due to inappropriate tooth movements, and the dento-alveolar changes associated with continued facial growth, it is perhaps fortunate that the post-retention changes in incisor relationship reported in many studies have been relatively small. When relapse is reported as statistically significant, it is often questionable whether the changes are of long term clinical significance.

With class III incisor relationships and where treatment is aimed at producing a positive overbite and overjet where they did not previously exist, the risk of relapse of the incisor relationship is high. It has been reported to be as great as 40 per cent when treatment is undertaken in the rapidly growing child.[24] Unfortunately there are no reliable predictors to indicate in which children the risk of relapse is high.[24,25] If there is any doubt over the long term stability of correction of a class III incisor relationship it is best to defer definitive treatment until facial growth has all but ceased (see Chapter 10).

9.4 ANTEROPOSTERIOR BUCCAL SEGMENT RELATIONSHIP

In an ideal occlusion, each upper tooth occludes with the corresponding lower arch tooth and the one distal to it, with the exception of the upper third permanent molar. In such a case the buccal segment relationship and, in particular, the molar relationship is described as class I (see Chapter 2). The same relationship applies in a normal occlusion. Indeed the attainment of a class I molar relationship is one of the fundamental 'six keys to normal occlusion'[26] and as such is a major treatment goal in cases being treated with the preadjusted edgewise fixed appliance system, more commonly known as the Straight-Wire® ('A' Company) system. However, in some cases treatment dictates the attainment of a different molar relationship. This can still provide full interdigitation of the buccal segment teeth but with the molar relationship being class II or less often class III. In some cases it is not possible to achieve full interdigitation and the buccal segment teeth will occlude in a position somewhere between class I and either class II or class III at the end of treatment. The importance of full buccal segment interdigitation and, in particular, a class I molar relationship has, however, been highlighted in a study on untreated occlusions in individuals from their late teenage years up to between 50 and 60 years of age.[27] It was found that 100 per cent of individuals who initially presented with a class I molar relationship still had this molar relationship 30–40 years later. Individuals who initially presented with class II and class III molar relationships, however, displayed a tendency for the molar relationship to deteriorate over the same time period, that is, become more class II or class III. Although the change in both cases was found to be statistically significant, the average measured change was small, being only 0.8 mm in the class II cases and 1.2 mm in the Class III cases. A subsequent investigation on orthodontic patients examined, on average, some 15 years post-retention has also demonstrated the improved stability conferred by full buccal segment tooth interdigitation.[28] In this case, the presence of full interdigitation, that is class I, II or III was associated with improved stability in terms of tooth alignment post-retention. In those cases where the molar relationship was somewhere between class I, II, and III at the end of treatment, there was an increased tendency to post-retention crowding and incisor irregularity.

9.5 ANTERIOR OPEN BITES

The aetiology of anterior open bites can include skeletal factors, such as an increased anterior lower face height; soft tissue factors, such as the tongue or lips interposing between the upper and lower incisors; or digit sucking habits. In the case of the latter an anterior open bite will often improve to some degree, particularly in the growing child, following cessation of the habit. Spontaneous closure of the open bite will be a good indicator of long term stability. By contrast, large anterior open bites due to skeletal causes may be outside the realms of orthodontic treatment, and a combined orthodontic and orthognathic approach may be appropriate.

For cases that are intermediate between these two extremes and where treatment will entail some extrusion of incisor teeth the following questions need to be considered before planning treatment.

1. How stable will the open bite correction be?
2. Will the alveolar bone follow the extrusion of the incisor teeth so there is no loss of bony support?
3. If relapse does occur, will any loss of alveolar bone support induced by tooth extrusion be regained if the incisors subsequently undergo some spontaneous intrusion?

Work performed at the University of Washington, Seattle has considered the long term stability of anterior open bite correction.[29] In a study on patients who had undergone orthodontic treatment for an anterior open bite of at least 3 mm, 35 per cent were found to demonstrate relapse when re-examined some $9\frac{1}{2}$ years post-retention. Relapse was defined as the reappearance of a 3 mm anterior open bite and so an even greater percentage of patients will exhibit some form of relapse of the original anterior open bite post-retention. Those patients with open bites of greater than 0 mm but less than 3 mm were not included in the relapse group. Lower incisor irregularity was also measured throughout the study and a significant degree of post-retention relapse was found in most cases, similar to that reported following orthodontic treatment of malocclusions other than anterior open bites.[13] What also would have been interesting to know is whether upper incisor irregularity post-retention was more marked in relapsed anterior open bite cases. With no vertical incisor overlap post-retention, it might also be expected to increase. For example, if the upper lateral incisor teeth had been palatally positioned prior to treatment of the anterior open bite, then relapse of the open bite might be expected to be accompanied by palatal relapse of the upper lateral incisors.

Orthodontic treatment of anterior open bites usually entails some extrusion of the incisor teeth to produce a positive overbite. As there are no positive predictors of relapse and since the likelihood of relapse is high, it is important to know whether incisor extrusion, followed by possible intrusion as the case relapses, is going to be detrimental to the long term health of the teeth or their supporting tissues. A limited study on root length, root morphology, and labial alveolar bone height has been performed on pre and post-treatment anterior open bite and increased overbite cases. Although prior to treatment the individuals with an anterior open bite were found to possess shorter upper incisor roots with less labial bony support than the increased overbite group, reassuringly the loss of root tissue and bony support as a result of treatment was found to be the same in both groups.[30] However, what is still unknown is whether those cases which undergo post-retention relapse of the open bite, probably by incisor intrusion, will suffer further damage to the roots and their supporting tissues as a result.

9.6 TRANSVERSE BUCCAL SEGMENT RELATIONSHIP

Just as changes in the labiolingual position of the lower incisors tend to relapse postretention, if the dental arch is expanded in order to create space for tooth alignment, there is a tendency for it to return towards its pretreatment width following retention. This has been shown to take place regardless of the length of the retention period post-treatment.[31] Subsequent to this relapse, there will be an increase in incisor crowding. An exception to this arch expansion relapse tendency will be the unilateral posterior crossbite with an associated displacement on closing into centric occlusion. Treatment by arch expansion to eliminate this displacement is likely to remain stable in the long term provided there is sufficient vertical cuspal overlap of the buccal segment teeth once treatment is complete. Rapid maxillary expansion (Fig. 9.3) is recommended by some as a means of eliminating bilateral posterior crossbites and creating space to align maxillary arch teeth. With this more aggressive form of arch expansion there is a large tendency to relapse, being in the region of 55 per cent in intermolar width and 77 per cent of intercanine width post-retention.[32] Even if the dental arch is not purposefully expanded as part of orthodontic treatment, arch form is commonly altered during treatment, especially when using modern fixed appliances with their preadjusted brackets and preformed arch wires. It seems that the arch will return towards its pretreatment form once all retaining appliances have been removed.[33] If care is taken to ensure that dental arch width and form are not changed during orthodontic treatment, there is still no guarantee that arch length and intercanine width will not decrease with age, and thus incisor alignment

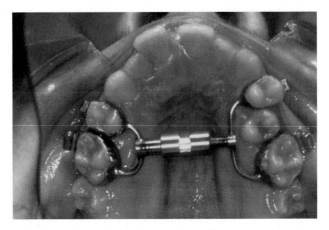

Fig. 9.3 Rapid maxillary expansion can be achieved using a midline screw cemented to the buccal segment teeth and activated twice a day for 10–14 days.

deteriorate. Such age variations should be considered as normal physiological changes which will consequently occur in both treated and untreated individuals.

9.7 ROTATED TEETH

Orthodontic correction of rotated teeth is straightforward, especially with fixed appliances, provided there is sufficient space within the arch for derotation to occur. However, as with many aspects of orthodontic treatment, the prediction of likely rotational relapse is more problematic than the treatment. The precise cause of rotational relapse is unknown but may be related to stretch in the supracrestal (transeptal and free gingival) fibres surrounding the derotated tooth[34] and possibly the principal fibres of the periodontium. The latter, however, have been shown to undergo remodelling within only 2–3 months of the tooth derotation.[35,36] Indian ink markers, when placed within the gingivae, demonstrate how the gingivae and particularly the marginal gingivae are pulled in the direction of the derotation during orthodontic treatment.[37] Supracrestal fibres have been demonstrated histologically to remain in this distorted position for some considerable time post-treatment[34] and may be responsible for the increased likelihood of post-treatment rotational relapse. As with other forms of orthodontic relapse, the amount observed is not usually related to the degree of preceding tooth movement (i.e. derotation) during treatment.[38] Methods which have been suggested to help minimize rotational relapse include

(1) early correction of the rotation after tooth eruption;

(2) over-correction of the rotation;

(3) prolonged retention;

(4) ensuring the correct interdigitation of opposing teeth; and

(5) pericision.

Unfortunately, none of the above can guarantee to prevent rotational relapse. The aim of pericision is to cut the supracrestal fibres around a derotated tooth and thereby lessen any effect these tissues might have on long term rotational stability. Indian ink markers within the gingivae have been demonstrated to return to their pretreatment position within 40 hours of this minor surgical procedure being performed.[38,39] In addition, the long term health effects on the periodontium are minimal. A notable exception to this, however, will be the labial gingivae around the lower incisors where there is a risk that pericision could lead to the creation of a dehiscence. This is a particular risk where the alveolar bone and gingival tissues overlying the labial aspect of these teeth can be very thin. Although pericision will help reduce rotational relapse in some instances, particularly in the upper incisor region, it has been found to be less effective in preventing rotational relapse in the case of the lower incisors. This is thought to be due to the multifactorial nature of the relapse mechanism in this part of the mouth.[39]

9.8 THE THIRD PERMANENT MOLARS

Two questions are commonly of importance in treatment planning in orthodontics with respect to the third permanent molars.

1. If teeth are extracted further mesially within the arch as part of treatment, will there be sufficient room created for the third permanent molars to erupt into a functional position?

2. Will retained third permanent molars cause a deterioration in the alignment of the teeth within the arch after orthodontic treatment has been completed?

It would seem that following the extraction of first or second permanent molars the third permanent molars will invariably have sufficient room to move into the line of the arch[40] and may or may not require appliance therapy to facilitate this. Certainly, following the loss of the second permanent molar, the third molar may be able to erupt spontaneously into the line of the arch, although there is no guarantee it will erupt into a good position.[41] Suggested criteria for it to occur include the following.

1. The angulation of the third permanent molar to the long axis of the first permanent molar should be less than 30° (Fig. 9.4).

2. Extraction of the second permanent molar should coincide with full crown formation of the unerupted third permanent molar.

3. There should not be any space between the crown of the unerupted third permanent molar and the roots of the second permanent molar.[42]

In the case of first and second premolar extractions some space may be created for the eruption of the third permanent molars.[43,44] However, it is no guarantee that the latter teeth will have sufficient space into which to erupt, since much will depend on the degree of crowding in the rest of the arch and how much residual space remains at the end of treatment.

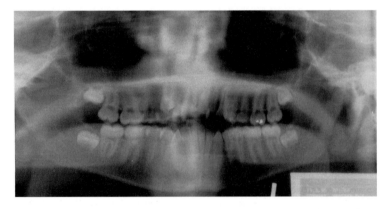

Fig. 9.4 Criteria when consideration is being given to the loss of second permanent molars: the third permanent molar should be present, of a good size and form; there must be no space between the unerupted third molar and the second molar; and the long axis of the third molar should be no more than 30° to the long axis of the first permanent molar.

Many papers have been written on the subject of the third permanent molars and late lower incisor crowding. In a comprehensive review of the literature[45] only a very limited and clinically insignificant link was found between the third molar and late lower incisor crowding. Subsequent work on subjects who underwent orthodontic treatment and who were at least 10 years post-retention demonstrated no differences in late lower incisor crowding between those who had third permanent molars and those who did not.[46] At present the loss of third permanent molars to prevent late lower incisor crowding is therefore not justified.

9.9 ROOT RESORPTION

During orthodontic tooth movement, it is usual for the alveolar bone in contact with the periodontium to undergo complex tissue remodelling wherever pressure is applied through the periodontal ligament to the bone (Fig. 9.5). This includes both activation of bone destruction by resorption and bone deposition. In this way, tooth movement can take place in the presence of an intact periodontium. At the same time, it is expected that the root of the tooth in question will remain intact. A possible reason for this is the presence of a protective layer where the periodontium meets the tooth, said to be composed of cementoblasts, fibroblasts, osteoblasts, and endothelial and perivascular cells.[47] An alternative protective layer is stated to be the cellular layer covering the root itself, namely the unmineralized layer of cementum or precementum.[48,49] Although a protective layer of one form or another is no doubt present, root resorption has been shown to occur when the force applied to the tooth causes the periodontium to undergo hyalinization.[49,50] This occurs when the force applied exceeds capillary blood pressure, and the compressed periodontal ligament assumes an avascular, glassy appearance under the microscope. Resorption begins between 10 and 35 days after force application and will cease when the force is reduced below capillary blood pressure. Subsequent repair takes place with the deposition of new cementum some 35–70 days after initial force application.[51,52] Up to 90.5 per cent of non-orthodontically treated teeth are thought to show microscopic signs of resorption.[48] Following orthodontic treatment, however, macroscopic signs of

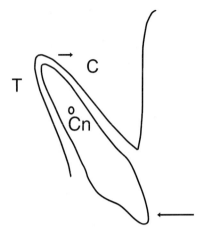

Fig. 9.5 Diagram illustrating the effect of tooth movement on the periodontal ligament and supporting bone during tooth movement. In this case the tooth has a load applied to rotate it about its centroid, (Cn). This classically establishes compression loads at C and tension loads at T. The former are said to promote bone loss while the latter promote bone deposition. There are many more theories relating mechanical load to the biological response, including (I) electrical causes such as piezoelectric and streaming potentials; (ii) biochemical causes including prostanoids and cytokines; (iii) mechanical load alone inducing stress and strain; and (iv) fluid flow such as occurs in the microcirculation.

resorption have been reported to be as high as 40 per cent in adults and 16.5 per cent in adolescents.[53] If radiographic evidence of resorption is seen during orthodontic treatment, it is recommended that treatment is ceased for 2–3 months, in order for repair to take place. Repair is in the form of a new layer of cementum being deposited in the previous area of resorption. Once repair has taken place, the risk of further root resorption on restarting treatment is then reduced, and overall the amount of root tissue lost will be reduced.[54] At the completion of orthodontic treatment, root resorption ceases, at least on a macroscopic scale.[55,56] If root resorption is so common, it would be useful to know if there are any predictors of those cases or teeth which are most likely to undergo a significant degree of resorption. An extensive review of the literature[57,58] examined many factors to determine whether there were any likely predictors of resorption. For many of the factors, the results of the review were inconclusive. The lack of a relationship between factors such as starting malocclusion, length of treatment, and type of appliance, for example, has been confirmed by more recent studies.[59,60] However, the following factors are of importance with respect to root resorption when planning orthodontic treatment.

1. Root form – blunt- or pipette-shaped roots show a greater susceptibility to resorption.

2. Pre-treatment root resorption – the presence of root resorption prior to orthodontic treatment is related to a higher prevalence of resorption post-treatment.

3. Habits – nail biting and endogenous tongue thrust are related to an increased risk of root resorption.

4. Age – root resorption is thought to occur more often in adults than in children and may be related to factors such as vascularity of the periodontium and bone density, that is, vascularity decreases and bone density increases with age.

5. Trauma – previously traumatized teeth with evidence of resorption are more prone to resorption during orthodontic treatment, whilst traumatized teeth without signs of resorption are not.

6. Root-treated teeth – these are thought to be less prone to resorption. This has been more recently confirmed in another study.[53] The reason a root filling confers some protection against resorption is related to the site of apical resorption. It is hypothesized that resorption occurs both on the external aspect of the root, closest to the periodontium, and on the pulpal aspect. A sound, well condensed, root filling will prevent apical resorption at this latter site.

9.10 TEMPOROMANDIBULAR JOINT DYSFUNCTION

Some of the possible iatrogenic effects of orthodontic treatment, such as damage to the teeth and their supporting tissues, which should be considered during diagnosis and treatment planning, have already been discussed in Chapter 7. Temporomandibular joint dysfunction with its varied signs and symptoms has also been suggested. The signs and symptoms can include palpable crepitus, audible clicking, pain in the joint which might radiate to the adjacent masticatory muscles, limitation of opening and sometimes trismus. It is a multi-factorial condition in which occlusal anomalies and orthodontic treatment have been suggested as two possible aetiological agents. In the United States an orthodontist was successfully sued by a patient who reportedly suffered temporomandibular joint dysfunction as a result of orthodontic treatment.[61] Following this legal action there has been a great deal of interest in the possible links between orthodontic treatment and temporomandibular joint dysfunction. Over 400 papers have been published on the subject[62] including extensive reviews of the available literature.[63,64,65] The following conclusions have been reached as a result of these works.

1. Intercuspal occlusal factors such as anterior open bite, increased overjet, increased overbite, or crossbites have a limited role in the aetiology of temporomandibular joint dysfunction.

2. Orthodontic treatment performed on children and adolescents is not a risk factor for the development of temporomandibular joint dysfunction in later life. This includes treatment with removable appliances, fixed appliances, both extraction and non-extraction treatment, the use of headgear, and also functional appliances.

3. The incidence of temporomandibular joint dysfunction in children and young adults tends to increase with age and as such may well develop during orthodontic treatment, but is not initiated by it.

4. Although orthodontic treatment is not implicated in the aetiology of temporomandibular joint dysfunction, neither should it be offered as a cure for the condition.

Summary of evidence based practice

Evidence based practice has four stated advantages.

1. It improves the effective use of research in clinical practice.
2. It enables more effective use of resources.
3. It produces less reliance on authority and more on evidence in clinical decision making.
4. It enables the practitioner to monitor and develop personal performance via audit or research.

Objectives

Understand the implications of the following with respect to orthodontic treatment.

1. Labiolingual positioning of the lower incisors
2. Lower incisor alignment
3. Correction of incisor relationship
4. Anteroposterior buccal segment relationship
5. Anterior open bites
6. Transverse buccal segment relationship
7. Rotated teeth
8. The third permanent molars
9. Root resorption
10. Temporomandibular joint dysfunction

REFERENCES

1. Richards, D. and Lawrence, A. (1995). Evidence based dentistry. *British Dental Journal*, **179**, 270–3.
2. Steiner, C. C. (1953). Cephalometrics for you and me. *American Journal of Orthodontics*, **39**, 729–55.
3. Tweed, C. H. (1969). The diagnostic facial triangle in the control of treatment objectives. *American Journal of Orthodontics*, **55**, 651–67.
4. Mills, J. R. E. (1966). The long term results of the proclination of the lower incisors. *British Dental Journal*, **120**, 355–63.
5. Mills, J. R. E. (1967). A long term assessment of mechanical retroclination of lower incisors. *Angle Orthodontist*, **37**, 165–74.
6. Williams, P. (1986). Lower incisor position in treatment planning. *British Journal of Orthodontics*, **13**, 33–41.
7. Downs, W. B. (1956). Analysis of dentofacial profile. *Angle Orthodontist*, **26**, 191–212.
8. Houston, W. J. B. and Edler, R. (1990). Long-term stability of the lower labial segment relative to the A–Pog line. *European Journal of Orthodontics*, **12**, 302–10.
9. Little, R. M. (1990). Stability and relapse of dental arch alignment. *British Journal of Orthodontics*, **17**, 235–41.
10. Kahl-Nieke, B., Fischbach, H., and Schwarze, C. W. (1996). Treatment and postretention changes in dental arch width dimensions – a long-term evaluation of influences cofactors. *American Journal of Orthodontics and Dento-Facial Orthopedics*, **109**, 368–78.

11. Weiland, F. J. (1994). The role of occlusal discrepancies in the long-term stability of the mandibular arch. *European Journal of Orthodontics*, **16**, 521–9.

12. Sinclair, P. M. and Little, R. M. (1983). Maturation of untreated normal occlusions. *American Journal of Orthodontics*, **83**, 114–23.

13. Little, R. M., Wallen, T. R., and Riedel, R. A. (1981). Stability and relapse of mandibular anterior alignment – first premolar extraction cases treated by traditional edgewise orthodontics. *American Journal of Orthodontics*, **80**, 349–65.

14. Little, R. M., Riedel, R. A., and Årtun, J. (1988). An evaluation of changes in mandibular anterior alignment from 10–20 years post-retention. *American Journal of Orthodontics and Dentofacial Orthopedics*, **93**, 423–8.

15. Björk, A. and Skieller, V. (1972). Facial development and tooth eruption. An implant study at the age of puberty. *American Journal of Orthodontics*, **62**, 339–83.

16. Houston, W. J. B. (1988). Mandibular growth rotations–their mechanisms and importance. *European Journal of Orthodontics*, **10**, 369–73.

17. Little, R. M. and Riedel, R. A. (1989). Postretention evaluation of stability and relapse – mandibular arches with generalised spacing. *American Journal of Orthodontics and Dentofacial Orthopedics*, **95**, 37–41.

18. Uhde, M. D., Sadowsky, C., and BeGole, E. (1984). Long-term stability of dental relationships after orthodontic treatment. *Angle Orthodontist*, **53**, 240–52.

19. Paquette, D. E., Beattie, J. R., and Johnston, L. E. (1992). A long-term comparison of nonextraction and premolar extraction edgewise therapy in 'borderline' Class II patients. *American Journal of Orthodontics and Dentofacial Orthopedics*, **102**, 1–14.

20. Sadowsky, C., Schneider, B. J., BeGole, E. A., and Tahir, E. (1994). Long-term stability after orthodontic treatment: nonextraction with prolonged retention. *American Journal of Orthodontics and Dentofacial Orthopedics*, **106**, 243–9.

21. Fidler, B. C., Årtun, J., Joondeph, D. R., and Little, R. M. (1995). Long-term stability of Angle class II, division 1 malocclusions with successful occlusal results at end of active treatment. *American Journal of orthodontics and Dentofacial orthopedics*, **107**, 276–85.

22. Drage, K. J. and Hunt, N. P. (1990). Overjet relapse following functional appliance therapy. *British Journal of Orthodontics*, **17**, 205–13.

23. Binda, S. K. R., Kuijpers-Jagtman, A. M., Maertens, J. K. M., and van't Hof, A. A. (1994). A long-term cephalometric evaluation of treated Class II division 2 malocclusions. *European Journal of Orthodontics*, **16**, 301–8.

24. Battagel, J. M. (1994). Predictors of relapse in orthodontically-treated Class III malocclusions. *British Journal of Orthodontics*, **21**, 1–13.

25. Stensland, A., Wisth, P. J., and Böe, O. E. (1988). Dentofacial changes in children with negative overjet treated by a combined orthodontic and orthopaedic approach. *European Journal of Orthodontics*, **10**, 39–51.
26. Andrews, L. F. (1972). The six keys to normal occlusion. *American Journal of Orthodontics*, **62**, 296–309.
27. Harris, E. F. and Behrents, R. G. (1988). The intrinsic stability of Class I molar relationship: a longitudinal study of untreated cases. *American Journal of Orthodontics and Dentofacial Orthopedics*, **94**, 63–7.
28. Kahl-Nieke, B., Fischbach, H., and Schwarze, C. W. (1995). Post-retention crowding and incisor irregularity: a long-term follow-up evaluation of stability and relapse. *British Journal of Orthodontics*, **22**, 249–57.
29. Lopez-Gavito, G., Wallen, T. R., Little, R. M., and Joondeph, D. R. (1985). Anterior open-bite malocclusion: a longitudinal 10-year postretention evaluation of orthodontically treated patients. *American Journal of Orthodontics*, **87**, 175–86.
30. Harris, E. and Butler M. L. (1992). Patterns of incisor root resorption before and after orthodontic correction in cases with anterior open bites. *American Journal of Orthodontics and Dentofacial Orthopedics*, **101**, 112–19.
31. Schwarze, C. W. (1972). Expansion and relapse in long follow-up studies. *Transactions of the European Orthodontic Society*, 263–74.
32. Linder-Aronson, S. and Lindgren, J. (1979). The skeletal and dental effects of rapid maxillary expansion. *British Journal of Orthodontics*, **6**, 25–9.
33. De La Cruz, R., Sampson, P., Little R. M., Årtun, J., and Shapiro, P. A. (1995). Long-term changes in arch form after orthodontic treatment and retention. *American Journal of Orthodontics and Dentofacial Orthopedics*, **107**, 518–30.
34. Reitan, K. (1959). Tissue rearrangement during retention of orthodontically rotated teeth. *Angle Orthodontist*, **29**, 105–13.
35. Reitan, K. (1958). Experiments on rotation of teeth and their subsequent retention. *Transactions of the European Orthodontic Society*, 124–40.
36. Deporter, D. A., Svoboda, E. L., Howley, T. P., and Shiga, A. (1984). A quantitative comparison of collagen phagocytosis in periodontal ligament and transeptal ligament of the rat periodontium. *American Journal of Orthodontics*, **85**, 519–22.
37. Edwards, J. G. (1968). A study of the periodontium during orthodontic rotation of teeth. *American Journal of Orthodontics*, **54**, 441–61.
38. Edwards, J. G. (1970). A surgical procedure to eliminate rotational relapse. *American Journal of Orthodontics*, **57**, 35–46.
39. Edwards, J. G. (1988). A long-term prospective evaluation of the circumferential supracrestal fiberotomy in alleviating orthodontic

relapse. *American Journal of Orthodontics and Dentofacial Orthopedics*, **93**, 380–7.

40. Richardson, M. E. (1975). The relative effects of the extraction of various teeth on the development of the third permanent molars. *Transactions of the European Orthodontic Society*, 79–85.

41. Cryer, B. S. (1967). Third molar eruption and the effect of extraction of adjacent teeth. *The Dental Practitioner*, **17**, 405–18.

42. Lawlor, J. (1978). The effects on the lower third molar of the extraction of the lower second molar. *British Journal of Orthodontics*, **5**, 99–103.

43. Richardson, M. E. (1989). The role of the third molar in the cause of late lower arch crowding: a review. *American Journal of Orthodontics and Dentofacial Orthopedics*, **95**, 79–83.

44. Richardson, M. E. (1989). The effect of mandibular first premolar extraction on third molar space. *Angle Orthodontist*, **59**, 291–4.

45. Vasir, N. S. and Robinson, R. J. (1991). The mandibular third molar and late crowding of the mandibular incisors – a review. *British Journal of Orthodontics*, **18**, 59–66.

46. Ades, A., Joondeph, D. R., Little, R. M., and Chapko, M. K. (1990). A long-term study of the relationship of third molars to changes in the mandibular dental arch. *American Journal of Orthodontics and Dentofacial Orthopedics*, **97**, 323–35.

47. Andreasen, J. O. (1988). A review of root resorption systems and models. Aetiology of root resorption and the homeostatic mechanisms of the periodontal ligament. In *Biological mechanisms of tooth eruption and root resorption*. EBSCO Media, Alabama (ed. Z. Davidovitch), pp. 9–22.

48. Henry, J. L. and Weinnmann, J. P. (1951). The pattern of resorption and repair of human cementum. *Journal of the American Dental Association*, **42**, 270–90.

49. Rygh, P. (1977). Orthodontic root resorption studied by electron microscopy. *Angle Orthodontist*, **47**, 1–16.

50. Reitan, K. (1974). Initial tissue behaviour during apical root resorption. *Angle Orthodontist*, **44**, 68–82.

51. Stenvik, A. and Mjör, I. A. (1970). Pulp and dentine reactions to experimental tooth intrusion. A histologic study of the initial changes. *American Journal of Orthodontics*, **57**, 370–85.

52. Harry, M. R. and Sims, M. R. (1982). Root resorption in bicuspid intrusion: a scanning electron microscope study. *Angle Orthodontist*, **52**, 235–58.

53. Mirabella, A. D. and Årtun, J. (1995). Prevalence and severity of apical root resorption of maxillary anterior teeth in adult orthodontic patients. *European Journal of Orthodontics*, **17**, 93–9.

54. Levander, E., Malmgren, O., and Eliasson, S. (1994). Evaluation of root resorption in relation to two orthodontic treatment regimes. A clinical experimental study. *European Journal of Orthodontics*, **16**, 223–8.

55. Copeland, S. and Green, L. J. (1986). Root resorption in maxillary central incisors following active orthodontic treatment. *American Journal of Orthodontics*, **89**, 51–5.

56. Remington, D., Joondeph, D. R., Årtun, J., Riedel, R. A., and Chapko, M. K. (1989). Long term evaluation of root resorption occurring during orthodontic treatment. *American Journal of Orthodontics and Dentofacial Orthopedics*, **96**, 43–6.

57. Brezniak, N. and Wasserstein, A. (1993). Root resorption after orthodontic treatment: Part 1. Literature review. *American Journal of Orthodontics and Dentofacial Orthopedics*, **103**, 62–6.

58. Brezniak, N. and Wasserstein, A. (1993). Root resorption after orthodontic treatment: Part 2. Literature review. *American Journal of Orthodontics and Dentofacial Orthopaedics*, **103**, 138–46.

59. Mirabella, A. D. and Årtun, J. (1995). Risk factors for apical root resorption of maxillary anterior teeth in adult orthodontic patients. *American Journal of Orthodontics and Dentofacial Orthopedics*, **108**, 48–55.

60. Blake, M., Woodside, D. G., and Pharoah, M. J. (1995). A radiographic comparison of apical root resorption after orthodontic treatment with edgewise and Speed appliances. *American Journal of Orthodontics and Dentofacial Orthopedics*, **108**, 76–84.

61. Pollack, B. (1988). Case of note: Michigan jury awards $850 000 in ortho case: a tempest in a teapot. *American Journal of Orthodontics and Dentofacial Orthopedics*, **94**, 358–9.

62. Behrents, R. G. and White, R. A. (1992). TMJ Research: responsibility and risk. *American Journal of Orthodontics and Dentofacial Orthopedics*, **101**, 1–3.

63. Sadowsky, C. S. (1992). The risk of orthodontic treatment for producing temporomandibular mandibular disorders: a literature overview. *American Journal of Orthodontics and Dentofacial Orthopedics*, **101**, 79–83.

64. Seligman, D. A. and Pullinger, A. G. (1991). The role of intercuspal occlusal relationships in temporomandibular disorders: a review. *Journal of Craniomandibular Disorders and Facial and Oral Pain*, **5**, 96–106.

65. Tallents, R. H., Catania, J., and Sommers, E. (1991). Temporomandibular joint findings in pediatric populations and young adults: a critical review. *Angle Orthodontist*, **61**, 7–16.

10

Treatment planning

Treatment planning is the stage of orthodontics at which, in many cases, science is replaced by art. Operators determine what can be achieved, generally based on their own previous experience, with some individuals being able to produce treatment results that others are incapable of producing with precisely the same facilities. To this end, many controversies exist in orthodontics which can only be alluded to in a text of this nature. It is important, however, to be aware that many debates as to the effectiveness of a particular mode of treatment often have little or no basis in scientific fact. Current controversies in orthodontic treatment planning include:

(1) extraction versus non-extraction treatments in the permanent dentition;

(2) whether to use headgear in view of the potential risk of eye injury;[1]

(3) the effect of orthodontic treatment on facial growth; and

(4) the potential risk of developing temporomandibular joint disorders as a consequence of orthodontic treatment.

Whatever the controversies, the treatment plan chosen for a particular case should have clearly defined and realistic treatment objectives. The four principal objectives are:

(1) to improve aesthetics (this is the major indication for performing orthodontic treatment);

(2) to produce a stable occlusal result (as discussed in Chapter 9, stability is often elusive and the patient needs to be made aware of this prior to starting any proposed treatment. Therefore, where possible, treatment planning should be based on meeting the patient's needs. Where this is not possible, the

reason(s) why should be fully explained to the patient before embarking on treatment of any kind);

(3) to improve dental health (see Chapter 7);

(4) to improve oral function.

In treatment planning it is important to understand that creation of an ideal class I incisor relationship, complete with 32 teeth in perfect occlusion, is an ideal which is seldom achieved.[2] This applies equally to the concept of the 'six keys' of an ideal occlusion. In some instances there may be a conflict of interest as to what should and can be achieved with orthodontic treatment. For example, in a case with drifting teeth due to periodontal involvement, orthodontic treatment without correction of the underlying periodontal condition would severely compromise dental health. In such circumstances the following order of priority should ideally be given in treatment planning:

(1) health

(2) stability

(3) aesthetics.

However, this order sometimes has to be modified. Using the same periodontal drifting example, dental health will be improved by treating the periodontal disease and if the tooth is left in its present position it will be in a state of balance with the soft tissues and remain stable. Orthodontic correction will undoubtedly improve aesthetics, but the corrected position is rarely stable and permanent retention is usually required.

It is always helpful when planning a case to devise a range of treatment plans from which the most appropriate can be chosen for the patient in question. These should range from the complex and usually ideal treatment plan, through to the simplest, usually a compromise plan. The following factors will influence the final choice between a simple or complex treatment approach to the management of a malocclusion:

1. Patient suitability (e.g. standard of oral hygiene and likely compliance).

2. Dento-alveolar factors (e.g. absence, ectopic position, or poor prognosis of teeth which may prevent the attainment of ideal occlusal relationships).

3. Skeletal pattern. Where the anteroposterior or vertical skeletal relationships are severe, the ideal treatment plan might require a combination of orthodontics and orthognathic surgery. However, surgery and the accompanying anaesthetic are not without risk, and a risk/benefit analysis might deem such treatment inappropriate. This might be accentuated if the patient has a complex medical history. In such circumstances it would be more appropriate to limit treatment to orthodontic alignment, without correction of the incisor relationship, followed by prolonged retention. Growth also needs to be considered.

4. Soft tissue pattern. This will have an influence on the long and short term stability of treatment. For example, in a class II division 1 incisor relationship an idealized treatment plan will be based on the assumption that any adaptive anterior oral seal will change following orthodontic treatment. However, should an underlying abnormal swallowing pattern persist, or if there is a failure of the lower lip to control the upper incisor position at the end of treatment, stability will be adversely affected. In such cases a compromise treatment plan may have to be considered, with limited objectives in terms of correction of the incisor relationship.

5. The patient's principal complaint. If a patient is concerned by the position of one particular tooth and there are no dental health or functional problems with the occlusion, it may be possible simply to align this tooth orthodontically and accept any minor tooth malalignments elsewhere. However, if the patient is concerned with the alignment of one tooth and yet there are potential dental health or functional implications elsewhere in the arch, then a more idealized plan will be required which should be explained fully to the patient.

6. The availability of clinical expertise. This will include not only the availability of orthodontic expertise, but also the availability of specialist support for complex treatments such as implants, restorative treatment, or orthognathic surgery.

It is important to realize that only the basic principles of treatment planning can be outlined in this book. In general, when planning orthodontic treatment, the lower arch should be considered first as the basis around which the upper arch can be positioned. This is mainly the case in class I and class II incisor relationships.

The anteroposterior and transverse dimensions of the lower arch should not be altered by orthodontic treatment, although crowding can be relieved and the teeth realigned within it. There are specific exceptions to this rule, particularly with respect to the anteroposterior positioning of the lower incisors, including

(1) class III incisor relationships where a deep overbite will maintain any changes in incisor inclination (i.e. retroclination of the lower incisors to produce a positive overjet);

(2) bimaxillary proclination cases where both upper and lower labial segments are to be retracted, and where incompetent lips can become competent;

(3) class II division 2 incisor relationships where both the upper and lower labial segments are retroclined as a consequence of adverse soft tissue behaviour;

(4) class II division 1 incisor relationships where there is a deep and complete overbite, usually to the palate. In such cases the lower incisors are retroclined as the mandible continues to grow forwards. The lower labial segment teeth are 'trapped' in the palate as normal development occurs;

(5) class II division 1 incisor relationships caused by a thumb or digit sucking habit. Cessation of the habit, often coincidental with active treatment, will allow the lower incisors to procline.

Most of the above exceptions not only require complex specialist treatment but also specialist diagnosis, supported by a cephalometric analysis. Such specialist assessment will often be required during and after orthodontic treatment not only to monitor progress, but also to try to determine the likely post-treatment stability.

The majority of orthodontic treatment is commenced in the late mixed or the early permanent dentition. However, adult patients are also becoming increasingly aware of the capabilities and potential benefits of orthodontic treatment. In such cases there is often a need for treatment to be combined with that from other specialist disciplines such as restorative dentistry and oral surgery.

10.1 THE TIMING OF ORTHODONTIC TREATMENT

When planning orthodontic treatment, the options available to the orthodontist, once active treatment is deemed appropriate, include

(1) tooth extraction only (i.e. without appliance therapy);

(2) the use of removable appliances, with or without extractions;

(3) the use of fixed appliances, with or without extractions;

(4) use of functional appliances which may or may not be followed by fixed appliance therapy (with or without extractions);

(5) orthognathic surgery concurrent with fixed appliance therapy.

The timing of such treatment modalities will depend not only on the malocclusion but obviously also on the developmental stage of the dentition, as listed below.

1. The deciduous dentition. Whereas active appliance therapy is not recommended at this stage, it is sometimes necessary to consider balancing and, less often, compensating extractions in order to preserve the centre lines and buccal segment relationships, respectively.

2. The mixed dentition phase. During this stage the following treatments may be undertaken:

    (a) balancing and sometimes compensating extractions of both deciduous and permanent teeth, with or without a passive removable appliance to act as a space maintainer;

    (b) simple treatment, using a removable appliance to correct an anterior crossbite (i.e. procline an incisor tooth over the bite), or buccal segment expansion to eliminate a posterior crossbite;

    (c) complex treatment aimed at correcting a severe class II or class III malocclusion using techniques such as functional appliances or headgear.

3. The early permanent dentition. It is at this stage that the majority of orthodontic treatment is performed. Not only are the permanent teeth in the mouth, but patients are actively growing and treatment in the majority of cases is well tolerated. It is important to remember that, although at this stage of development patients are less prone to periodontal disease, they are more susceptible to dental caries, and this should be considered when planning any extractions. Treatment which involves extractions without appliances can only be undertaken when teeth adjacent to the chosen extraction sites are favourably angulated away from them. Removable appliances

are of use where simple tipping movements are required to align teeth and correct the incisor relationship. Fixed appliances will be necessary wherever bodily tooth movements are planned, or where multiple rotations require correction. Both appliance types may be used with or without extractions or headgear, as necessary. During the early permanent dentition phase, functional appliances are often used to help correct, in particular, moderate to severe class II skeletal and incisor relationships. This is most effective during the period of rapid facial growth associated with the pubertal growth 'spurt'.[3]

4.   The adult dentition stage. Treatment at this time can include removable or fixed appliance therapy, with or without extractions and sometimes in combination with orthognathic surgery. However, although orthodontic treatment in these patients is becoming commonplace, treatment in adulthood can present specific problems.

  (a)   There are no major growth changes, although the facial skeleton undergoes remodelling. This can make vertical occlusal changes, such as overbite reduction, very difficult. It also means that functional appliances are of little use in the correction of anteroposterior skeletal discrepancies.

  (b)   Following extractions, adjacent teeth will undergo only a limited amount of spontaneous movement. If active tooth movement is not undertaken, the alveolus in the extraction site will resorb, giving it a wasted appearance. Subsequent orthodontic tooth movement into this area of resorbed alveolus can be very difficult, if not impossible. Anteriorly, a wasted alveolus can also pose an aesthetic problem.

  (c)   The blood supply to the alveolar bone and dental structures in adults is functionally less than in teenage patients.[4] This has two major consequences. First, the products of inflammation can build up rapidly leading to more frequent pain of a longer duration during orthodontic tooth movement. Second, the lack of perfusion can put dental structures at risk, particularly the alveolar bone and dental pulp, leading to possible bone loss and pulpal death.

  (d)   The pattern of dental disease is different in adult patients. In particular they are more susceptible to periodontal disease. Not only can alveolar bone loss modify the response to normal 'orthodontic' levels of loading, but the risk of active disease being exaggerated by the application of orthodontic tooth movement cannot be overlooked. Dental movement in the presence of inflammation will lead to a rapid and dramatic reduction in alveolar bone height.

These four developmental phases will now be dealt with in turn and, for convenience, the early permanent dentition and the adult dentition stages will be discussed together.

10.2 THE DECIDUOUS DENTITION

Orthodontic treatment is rarely indicated in this stage of development. However, it is sometimes necessary to consider deciduous tooth extractions when teeth elsewhere in the arch have been lost due to caries or trauma. Such planned treatments are known as balancing or compensating extractions and will be considered under the mixed dentition phase.

10.3 THE MIXED DENTITION PHASE

This developmental stage has been outlined in Chapter 1 and begins with the eruption of the first permanent molars and continues until eruption of the premolar teeth. Determination of a definitive long term treatment plan for the patient is often not possible at this time. Not only can the assessment of potential crowding or spacing within the dentition be difficult but, in some patients, particularly those with moderate class III skeletal patterns, it is difficult to estimate the long term effects of facial growth on the occlusion with any degree of certainty. However, it is possible to assist the development of the dentition by undertaking interceptive procedures. Such practices include balancing, compensating, and serial extractions and are aimed at simplifying later definitive treatment in the early permanent dentition.

10.3.1 Balancing extractions

These are performed in order to maintain the dental centre line and can include the loss of a deciduous canine or first deciduous molar to balance the loss of the same tooth on the opposite side of the same arch. The choice of tooth for the balancing extraction will often be dictated by its prognosis and condition, but in general the deciduous canine is the balancing extraction of choice. Second deciduous molar loss is never balanced by the loss of any contralateral tooth. This is because:

(1) the effect of second deciduous molar loss on the centre line is minimal; and

(2) a balancing extraction of the second deciduous molar on the opposite side of the same arch can lead to rapid space loss as a result of mesial movement of the first permanent molar.

10.3.2 Compensating extractions

These are carried out in opposing arches in order to maintain buccal segment relationships. They are not frequently performed.

10.3.3 Serial extractions

These were originally advocated by Kjellgren[5] with the stated aim of relieving crowding and allowing the development of an acceptable occlusion, without the need for extensive appliance treatment in the permanent dentition. The serial extraction regimen is:

(1) loss of the deciduous canines around $8\frac{1}{2}$ years of age, as the upper lateral incisors are erupting, in order to relieve permanent incisor crowding;

(2) loss of first deciduous molars one year later, in order to encourage the eruption of the first premolars in advance of the permanent canines;

(3) removal of the first premolars as the permanent canines are beginning to erupt, allowing the latter teeth into the line of the arch.

The classic case for serial extractions must have:

(1) a class I or a mild class II or III skeletal base;

(2) a class I incisor relationship; and

(3) all teeth present and in their normal developmental positions.

There are a number of problems with the serial extraction regimen.

1. In the lower arch there is no guarantee that extraction of the first deciduous molars will encourage the first premolars to erupt before the permanent canines.

2. In the upper arch, the first premolar will erupt before the permanent canine regardless of the deciduous molar extraction.

3. Rarely will a case meet all the correct criteria, such that following the extractions an ideal occlusion will be created without the need for appliance therapy.

4. The child must tolerate three phases of extractions, which may necessitate subjecting the child to three general anaesthetics.

It is for these reasons that the complete serial extraction regimen is of limited use. Instead, it is common for parts of it to be used and the rest of the regimen to be disregarded. For example, deciduous canines may be extracted to permit alignment of a lingually positioned and partially erupted lower incisor, or to permit alignment where one permanent incisor is so labially placed as to jeopardize its long term periodontal health. No further extractions may then be required. On the other hand, the first extractions undertaken as part of a patient's treatment may be the removal of the first premolars, in order to permit displaced and crowded canines to move into the arch. First deciduous molar extractions are never performed electively, unless the teeth are of poor prognosis and as part of a balancing extraction. Selective extractions in this manner in the mixed dentition can be considered as longitudinal guidance of the developing dentition.[6]

In addition to such longitudinal guidance, it is possible to commence active orthodontic treatment in the mixed dentition stage. However, this must be prudently undertaken in order to avoid extending the overall treatment time and overburdening the patient's compliance. This is particularly so if further active orthodontic treatment may be required in the permanent dentition. The types of treatment undertaken in the mixed dentition stage are described in the following sections.

10.3.4 Correction of crossbites

Generally, correction of a crossbite should take no longer than 4–6 months and is easily performed using a removable appliance.

Before embarking upon treatment it is important to determine whether there is a displacement on closing into centric occlusion. In the case of anterior crossbites, three further features should be assessed:

(1) the depth of the overbite – a positive overbite must be present post-treatment in order to provide a stable occlusal result;

(2) the anteroposterior skeletal pattern – ideally this should be class I or only mild class III;

(3) the inclination of the upper and lower incisors – ideally, the upper incisors should be slightly retroclined so that following their proclination to eliminate the crossbite they will be at the correct inclination post-treatment. The lower incisors should be of average inclination or slightly proclined. If the opposite is true, namely proclined upper incisors and retroclined lower incisors at the start of treatment, then dento-alveolar compensation is present in combination with the class III skeletal pattern. Correction of the crossbite in this case, even in the presence of a displacement and a positive overbite, may lead to excessive proclination of the upper incisors with resultant unfavourable loading of the teeth in function.

In the case of posterior crossbites, in addition to a displacement, there should be a positive occlusal 'interlock' following upper arch expansion. The transverse skeletal relationships should ideally be normal, with little in the way of dento-alveolar compensation (i.e. the upper cheek teeth should not be particularly buccally inclined nor the lowers particularly lingually inclined as a result of a transverse skeletal discrepancy). Patients with a flat cuspal morphology, often as a consequence of wear, will have a tendency towards the relapse of upper arch expansion. Posterior crossbites with a displacement are usually unilateral and rarely bilateral.

At this same mixed dentition stage of occlusal development, a child may be encouraged to give up a persistent digit sucking habit by the use of a simple upper removable appliance. This same appliance can then be used to expand the upper arch if there is an associated unilateral crossbite with a displacement. However, care should be taken to ensure that the habit ceases prior to active expansion if the corrected crossbite is to remain stable. It should be remembered that a child can easily remove such an appliance in order to indulge in the habit, which if present on completion of treatment, will lead to almost certain relapse. Ideally the patient should cease the habit by other means before any appliances are fitted for active orthodontic treatment. In some cases reasoned explanation can result in stopping the habit if the child is eager to stop. Certain signs, however, such as a habit that occurs at night or undue parental pressure to cease the habit, are often indicators of a poor prognosis.

10.3.5 Functional appliance therapy

Functional appliances are used principally for the correction of moderate to severe class II division 1 incisor relationships on moderate to severe class II skeletal bases. They are less often used in the correction of class III incisor relationships on moderate to severe class III skeletal bases, due to a much lower success rate. The aim of carrying out this type of treatment at this stage is to maximize changes in facial growth, adaptation, and development. The appliance should be fitted just prior to the pubertal growth spurt (approximately 10–11 years of age in girls and 12–13 years in boys)[3] in order to ensure that it is in place during the most rapid period of growth. Treatment success is extremely difficult to predict. Both the appliance and patient require skilled handling and management if success is to be achieved. A cephalometric analysis should be performed at the beginning and end of treatment in order that treatment changes can be assessed and the likely stability of the final result predicted. Such treatments are principally performed by specialists in orthodontics who not only have the appropriate skills, but also the necessary support, particularly laboratory and radiographic.

10.4 THE EARLY PERMANENT DENTITION AND THE ADULT DENTITION STAGES

This stage of development is when most treatment is performed, because:

(1) the assessment of crowding or spacing is more easily and accurately made following the eruption of the majority of the permanent dentition;

(2) facial growth is still occurring, which will assist tooth movement, particularly overbite reduction;

(3) most patients are compliant. Not only is treatment with appliances well tolerated, but the patient is usually able to understand the rationale both for treatment and appliance use;

(4) treatment can usually be completed within an acceptable time scale of 18–24 months.

It must be remembered that whilst the general characteristics of facial form have developed at this age, further growth is yet to take place. Although there are no reliable mechanisms to predict the growth potential of an individual, it is usually safe to assume an average degree of facial growth. The relationship between the maxilla and the mandible will therefore change little with time. Exceptions to this include moderate to severe class III skeletal bases in which continued facial growth may lead to a worsening of the class III skeletal relationship.

In recent years it has been realized that different facial types can be classified, in addition to the more usual skeletal and incisor classifications. These facial types include the so-called high and low angle cases. In the former there is usually an increased anterior lower face height and Frankfort–mandibular planes angle. Intra-orally the overbite may be reduced, with extreme cases demonstrating an anterior open bite. In the low angle cases the opposite is true. The importance of recognizing such facial types lies in understanding the facial growth that has created the facial form and how such growth is likely to continue. Generally, a patient with the high angle face demonstrates a posterior growth rotation of the mandible, while a patient with a low angle face will have an anterior growth rotation of the mandible. Such growth rotations not only create these facial forms, but with time may make them more pronounced, especially if the mechanics of orthodontic treatment do not attempt to prevent this trend. Growth rotations are really considered as a mismatch of growth between the anterior and posterior facial heights. Some of the characteristic features of posterior and anterior growth rotators have already been alluded to, but further radiographic features seen on a lateral skull radiograph include:

(1) posterior mandibular growth rotation (Fig. 10.1):
    (a) a concave lower border of the mandible

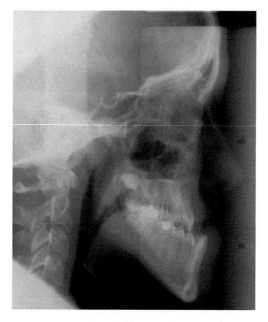

Fig. 10.1 The typical appearance of the mandible in a posterior growth rotation. Notice the concave lower border of the mandible.

    (b) an almost straight inferior dental nerve canal
    (c) a backwards slanting inner cortex of the mandible
    (d) a backwards inclined head of the condyle relative to ramus;
(2) anterior mandibular growth rotations (Fig. 10.2):
    (a) a convex lower border of the mandible
    (b) the inferior dental nerve canal forms almost a right angle at the ramus
    (c) a forwards slanting inner cortex of the mandible
    (d) a forwards inclined head of the condyle.

Growth rotations not only affect facial form but also the mechanisms used in orthodontic treatment. These are particularly related to vertical alterations in the occlusion, where it is all too easy to make the malocclusion worse with inappropriate treatment mechanics. A patient presenting with an anterior growth rotation,

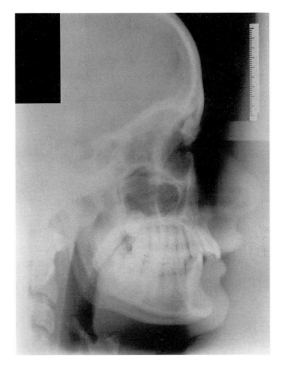

Fig. 10.2   The typical appearance of the mandible in an anterior growth rotation. Notice the convex lower border of the mandible.

typically a class II division 2 incisor relationship, should have treatment mechanics aimed at extruding the posterior teeth when reducing a deep overbite, to include

(1) removable and functional appliances, encouraging over-eruption of the lower buccal segment teeth by the use of a biteplane. The lower incisors are prevented from erupting by the action of the biteplane, whilst the posterior teeth are free to erupt. This biteplane effect can also be built into functional appliances by appropriate trimming of the acrylic overlying the lower posterior teeth. As the lower buccal segment teeth erupt, so the anterior lower face height may increase;

(2) fixed appliances. Extrusion of upper molars can be undertaken by using low- or cervical-pull headgear to bands cemented to

the upper molars. Extrusion of lower molars occurs using intra-oral elastics with fixed appliances.

Conversely, in posterior growth rotation, the treatment mechanics should aim to intrude the molars, using

(1) removable appliances and headgear: posterior biteplanes on an upper removable appliance in combination with high-pull headgear to the upper buccal segments;

(2) functional appliances. It is important that the posterior teeth are prevented from erupting by not trimming the interocclusal acrylic in the buccal segments. The Clark twin block is one such functional appliance which, in addition to the interocclusal blocks, has an anterior elastic in an attempt to promote anterior growth rotation;[7]

(3) fixed appliances. Once again, high pull headgear can be attached to the upper buccal segment teeth for intrusion.

Treatment planning will now be considered for each of the malocclusions in turn.

10.5 CLASS I MALOCCLUSIONS

Generally, in such cases, the skeletal and soft tissue patterns are favourable and close to normal. That is, the skeletal bases are related normally, one to the other, and the lips are competent at rest with no abnormal or adaptive soft tissue behaviour present. When planning treatment in a class I malocclusion the lower arch should be assessed first. The overall labiolingual position of the lower incisors and the intercanine and intermolar widths should all remain unaltered by orthodontic treatment, unless localized problems dictate otherwise. Treatment of the lower arch will depend upon the degree of spacing or crowding present.

10.5.1 Spaced lower arch

If there is spacing present, this should either be accepted or a lower fixed appliance will be required. In the latter case, the aims of treatment will either be to close the spacing, or if one or more teeth are developmentally absent, to relocate the spacing prior to provision of a prosthetic replacement.

10.5.2 Crowded lower arch

In this case a decision has to be made whether to accept it, if very mild, or to treat it via an extraction or non-extraction approach. If mild (less than 4 mm)[8] the crowding may be accepted and no appliances fitted. However, not uncommonly, a lower fixed appliance is used to align very mildly crowded teeth but it should be remembered that such treatment will lead to proclination of the lower incisors, away from a position of stability and into the lower lip. Following such treatment, it is usually necessary for the patient to wear a retainer for an indefinite period, either on a full or part time basis to prevent lower incisor relapse. Where mild to moderate crowding is present, a premolar unit is usually extracted on each side of the lower arch in order to relieve it. A space analysis will reveal whether this should be a first or second premolar. First premolar extractions usually provide more space, since these teeth are closer to the site of labial segment crowding. If crowding is to be relieved by lower second premolar loss, then more teeth need to be moved distally in order to enable the lower incisors to be aligned. Movement of more anterior teeth will increase the likelihood that the posterior teeth will move mesially, leading to greater anchorage loss (see Glossary). Overall, the amount of space provided by lower second premolar extractions will therefore be less as a result of a greater degree of mesial movement of the lower molar teeth. In performing a space analysis it is important not only to determine the amount of crowding in millimetres, but also to determine the type of tooth movement required to align the teeth. For spontaneous improvement in the alignment of the lower incisors following the loss of two lower first premolars, the lower canines should be angulated mesially away from the extraction sites. The lower incisors should either be angulated normally, or slightly mesially, with minimal or no rotations. If the lower canines or lower incisors are angulated distally and lower premolar loss is planned, then fixed appliances will be required to move the root apices distally. In addition the canines will have to be retracted and the incisors aligned. Such distal movement of the root apices will put a greater strain on the anchor teeth (i.e. the teeth distal to the extraction sites), increasing the possible risk of movement mesially into the extraction site. Such higher anchorage cases will therefore require more space and the extraction of first rather than second premolars is preferable. Sometimes the loss of first premolars will provide only

sufficient space to align the lower labial segment teeth, in which
case it is necessary to reinforce the lower arch anchorage by fitting
a lingual arch when using a fixed appliance. Very occasionally,
crowding in the lower labial segment, where both the lower
canines and lower incisors are distally angulated, can be relieved
by the loss of one lower incisor. Treatment usually requires fixed
appliances to ensure complete space closure and should only be
considered where

(1) the upper arch does not require treatment;
(2) the molar relationship is class I;
(3) following the lower incisor loss there will be complete space
     closure without an increase in the overjet or inducing crowd-
     ing in the upper labial segment.

10.5.3 Upper arch treatment

Once the lower arch treatment has been planned, the upper arch
should be considered. The aims of treatment will be to maintain a
class I incisor relationship, relieve crowding in the upper arch,
where present, and align the teeth. The key to treatment planning
in the upper arch lies in the position of the upper canine. For the
incisors to be aligned and in a class I relationship with the lower
incisors, the canine relationship must be corrected to class I. To
achieve this the following rules apply.

1. If the lower arch has been treated by the loss of a premolar unit
    in each quadrant then a premolar will need to be extracted in
    each quadrant in the upper arch. Depending upon the degree of
    crowding present in the upper arch, it may also be necessary to
    reinforce the anchorage by using headgear, or to create more
    space in the upper arch by distalizing the upper buccal segment
    teeth, prior to extracting a premolar unit in each quadrant. The
    final molar relationship must be class I if the canines and then
    the incisors are to be placed into a class I relationship.
2. If the lower arch has been accepted, because it is well-aligned
    or treated on a non-extraction basis, then the following options
    are available.
    (a) If the buccal segment relationship is half a unit class II or
         less (i.e. less than a premolar width of space is required to

move the canines into a class I relationship) the required space can be created by distalizing the upper buccal segment teeth using headgear to either a removable or fixed appliance. The final molar relationship will be class I.

(b) If the buccal segment relationship is more than a half a unit class II then a premolar should be extracted in each quadrant in the upper arch and the final molar relationship will be class II. The canine and incisor relationships will be class I.

(c) The closer the buccal segment relationship is to a full unit class II relationship prior to treatment, the greater the likelihood that headgear will be required to reinforce the anchorage in the upper arch. This is in addition to the loss of a premolar unit in each quadrant in the upper arch. If headgear is required, then the teeth of choice for extraction are the upper first premolars. It is a sign of incorrect diagnosis if upper second premolars are extracted and yet headgear has to be used, unless the latter teeth are extracted in preference to the first premolars due to a poorer prognosis (e.g. caries or periodontal disease). The final molar relationship will be class II, whilst the canine and incisor relationship will be class I.

(d) If the buccal segment relationship is already a full unit class II then headgear to reinforce the anchorage will be necessary from the start, in addition to the loss of a premolar unit in each upper quadrant. This will be necessary because the final molar relationship will be class II.

(e) Where the molar relationship is more than a full unit class II at the start, the upper buccal segment teeth need to be actively distalized using headgear, usually prior to upper first premolar loss, the latter teeth only being extracted once the molar relationship has been distalized to a full unit class II.

It can be seen that to produce a class I canine and incisor relationship the molar relationship can be either class I or class II, depending on the degree of crowding and the treatment mechanics chosen. Rarely is a class III molar relationship chosen as it would lead to excess spacing in the upper arch at the end of treatment.

Once space has been created in the upper arch, the choice between an upper removable or a fixed appliance to treat the malocclusion will depend on dental factors, such as the inclination and angulations of teeth and the number of rotations present. It should be remembered that removable appliances are only able to tip teeth about a point one third of the way down from the apex of the root.[9] Hence favourable teeth for movement with removable appliances are those angulated away from the created space. Wherever bodily tooth movement is required, or if there are multiple or marked rotations of teeth, then fixed appliances should be used.

10.6 CLASS II DIVISION 1 MALOCCLUSIONS

In the planning of treatment for class II division 1 malocclusions the aetiology of the malocclusion needs to be determined. If the malocclusion is due to a persistent digit sucking habit then the patient should be discouraged from the habit and the malocclusion reassessed six months later, when some spontaneous improvement should have occurred. Fortunately, purely soft tissue causes for this malocclusion are rare. Generally, the major determinant as to the type of treatment required is the presence or absence of a skeletal discrepancy.

10.6.1 No skeletal discrepancies

These are often assessed by the angles ANB and MMA. If there are no discrepancies, either anteroposterior or vertical, then treatment planning is similar to that outlined for class I malocclusions. Planning should begin in the lower arch, aiming to align the teeth and ideally closing any residual extraction spaces where present. The upper arch is then made to fit around the planned lower arch. The aim is not only to align the upper teeth but to move the canines and then the incisors into a class I relationship. The final molar relationship will depend upon the need for lower arch extractions and whether the upper arch is treated by extractions or distal movement. It should be remembered that the presence of an overjet is indicative of crowding, even when the teeth in the upper labial segment appear well aligned. At the end of treatment the stability of the incisor relationship will depend mainly on the presence of a lip to lip anterior oral seal at rest, with the incisal third of the upper incisor crowns being covered by the lower lip.

10.6.2 Skeletal discrepancy present

Vertical skeletal discrepancies with this malocclusion are usually high angle cases and as discussed previously, may show evidence of a posterior growth rotation of the mandible (see Fig. 10.1). Some of the problems in treating such cases have already been discussed, and relate not only to a possible worsening of the high angle during growth, but also to the long term stability of any correction. If the anterior lower face height is such that the lips are incompetent at the end of treatment, then it is likely the upper incisor correction will relapse. Fortunately, in most instances the skeletal discrepancy, when present, is anteroposterior, which from both the orthodontic and surgical points of view, is easier to treat than a vertical discrepancy. When the skeletal pattern is a mild class II, orthodontic treatment using removable or fixed appliances can be used to correct the malocclusion. As the skeletal pattern increases in severity, simple removable appliances, which tip the teeth, are of less value. Tipping the upper incisors to reduce an overjet in such instances can lead to over-retraction of the teeth and the creation of a class II division 2 incisor relationship. Fixed appliances will therefore be required, as they are able to retract teeth bodily, thereby creating a class I incisor relationship with the correct interincisal angle. As the anteroposterior skeletal relationship passes from mild to moderate and then to severe, even fixed appliances will be of limited use. Not only may there be insufficient bone palatal to the upper incisors for the teeth to be retracted (assessed from the lateral skull radiograph), but if the overjet were to be reduced purely by bodily retraction of the upper incisors, facial aesthetics may be compromised. This is because the principal aetiological agent in creation of this Class II division 1 incisor relationship is the moderate or severe skeletal class II relationship. Usually this is due to a retrognathic mandible.

10.6.3 Use of myofunctional appliances

In the growing patient, myofunctional appliances (e.g. bionator, Fig. 10.3; activator; Clark twin block) can be used to achieve an anteroposterior correction of the malocclusion. The appliances are fitted just before the start of the pubertal growth spurt and are worn during this period of rapid facial growth. The precise mode of action of such

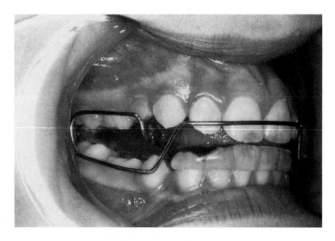

Fig. 10.3   An intra-oral photograph of a patient with a bionator in place.

appliances is somewhat controversial, but the principal modes of action may include dento-alveolar, skeletal, and soft tissue effects.

Dento-alveolar effects

These include:

- tipping of the upper incisors palatally;
- proclination of the lower incisors (usually an unwanted effect);
- a biteplane effect (lower incisor eruption is limited whilst permitting eruption of the posterior buccal segments);
- a distalizing effect on the upper buccal segment teeth. In combination with lower molar eruption in a mesial direction, the molar relationship may progress towards a class I from a class II;
- upper arch expansion by appropriate trimming of acrylic (bionator) or the use of a midline screw (Clark twin block).

Skeletal effects

These are extremely difficult to quantify because:

(1) the method of measurement may not be accurate enough to assess changes;

(2) the changes may not be permanent;

(3) the changes may occur during normal growth irrespective of therapy;

(4) patient compliance and actual skeletal age are variables that cannot be assessed accurately and so treatment success is difficult to establish.

The reported skeletal effects include:

• creating a larger mandible than would otherwise have occurred – very controversial;

• causing accelerated growth of the mandible and arresting growth in the maxilla during the period of wear of the appliance. The occlusion can then be corrected and dento-alveolar adaptation will maintain the occlusal result when the functional appliance is no longer worn. This is slightly less controversial;

• causing a change in direction of mandibular growth. This is the least controversial mode of action. For example, it is all too easy to make a high angle case worse by inappropriate use of a functional appliance, with the buccal segment teeth being allowed to continue to erupt.

Soft tissue effects

The premise that correction of the soft tissues in such cases will lead to correction of the malocclusion has been advocated by Fränkel,[10] but by few others. It is likely that Fränkel appliances work in the same manner as other myofunctional appliances in the correction of class II division 1 malocclusions.

When a myofunctional appliance is used to effect an anteroposterior change, both skeletal and dento-alveolar, the presence or absence of crowding can be ignored until the first or anteroposterior or sagittal phase of treatment is complete. If the teeth are well aligned at the start of treatment, then the malocclusion may just require treatment with the myofunctional appliance. However, where there is crowding or spacing superimposed on the class II division 1 incisor relationship, it is usual for the patient to undergo a subsequent or second phase of treatment using fixed appliances, after the myofunctional appliance phase. The precise planning of this second phase will be similar to that for a class I malocclusion with crowding or spacing, as described previously. The transition from the first myofunctional phase to the second fixed appliance phase can be difficult. This is particularly so with regards to the stability of the myofunctional phase of treatment, as well as the control of anchorage in the fixed appliance phase. Combined myofunctional and fixed appliance treatment is best undertaken by specialists in orthodontics.

Adult patients with a class II division 1 incisor relationship on a moderate to severe class II skeletal base will usually require a combined orthodontic and orthognathic approach to correct their malocclusion. The orthodontic treatment will be aimed at relief of crowding and alignment of the teeth using fixed appliances. The teeth, in particular the labial segment teeth, are decompensated so that the incisors are at the appropriate angle with respect to the maxillary and mandibular bases. Such decompensation then ensures the correct degree of mandibular or maxillary movement during surgery to rectify the underlying skeletal discrepancy. In the case of moderate to severe vertical skeletal discrepancies the combined orthodontic and surgical option may be the only means of correcting the malocclusion and creating a stable result. This is because the anterior lower face height can be reduced surgically, thereby enabling the patient to achieve a lip to lip anterior oral seal with sufficient coverage of the upper incisor crowns to retain their corrected position post-treatment.

10.7 CLASS II DIVISION 2 MALOCCLUSIONS

Whereas skeletal pattern has a major influence on treatment planning in class II division 1 malocclusions, in class II division 2 malocclusions the major determinant of treatment planning is whether the overbite can be accepted or not. Anteroposterior or vertical skeletal discrepancies, where present, are usually mild.

10.7.1 Overbite can be accepted

Although the overbite may be increased, if it is complete to tooth and therefore not traumatic to the gingivae of either the upper or lower incisors, it can be accepted. Certainly class II division 2 malocclusions are often aesthetically acceptable, both extra-orally and intra-orally, in which case it is perfectly reasonable to leave the malocclusion untreated. However, if there is crowding which requires treatment, then as is the case with class I and class II division 1 malocclusions, treatment planning should begin in the lower arch. A common complaint of patients with this malocclusion is not the increased overbite or any lower arch crowding, but the appearance of the proclined, mesially angulated, and mesiolabially rotated upper lateral incisors (Fig. 10.4). If lower arch crowding is very mild, it can be accepted and treatment can be aimed at aligning the upper lateral incisors to the same anteroposterior position as the upper central incisors. The necessary space can be created either by the loss of a premolar unit in each quadrant in the upper arch, or by distal movement of the upper buccal segment teeth. Often only a small amount of space is required, less than half a premolar width on each side of the upper arch, in which case distal movement using headgear is preferable to extractions which would create too much space. In performing distal movement, it is often not necessary to retract the upper molars and premolars to a class I buccal segment relationship with the corresponding lower arch teeth, otherwise the patient will end up with residual space, usually distal to the upper canines, at the end of treatment. The buccal

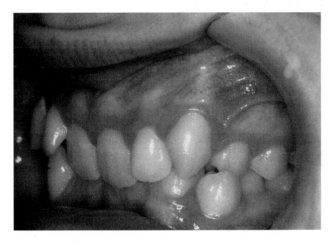

Fig. 10.4 A common complaint in a class II division 2 incisor relationship is not the deep overbite, but the proclined mesially angulated, and mesiolabially rotated upper lateral incisors. In this case the upper right lateral incisor is shown to be proclined.

segment teeth only need to be retracted sufficiently to create space for the retraction of the upper canines and alignment of the upper lateral incisors. All this treatment can be performed using upper removable appliances and headgear. The headgear will be used to actively retract the upper buccal segment teeth at first, using a force of 500 g per side with 12–14 hours of wear (extra-oral traction). During canine retraction and upper lateral incisor alignment, headgear wear can then be reduced to nights only, usually 8–10 hours of wear, with a force of only 250 g per side (extra-oral anchorage).

If there is sufficient crowding in the lower arch to warrant extractions for the relief of crowding, even though the pretreatment overbite is acceptable, then serious consideration should be given to the use of a lower fixed appliance. The reason for this is that extractions in the lower arch without fixed appliance therapy may lead to the lower labial segment teeth assuming a new aligned position which is retroclined to a greater degree than before. This slight lingual repositioning may be sufficient to transform a deep overbite, which is just complete to tooth, into a deep overbite which is traumatic and complete to the gingivae palatal to the upper incisors, or labial to the lower incisors. If a lower fixed appliance is to be used, then it is worth correcting the overbite and the interincisal angle with both a lower and an upper fixed appliance in order to create a class I incisor relationship, a good edge-centroid relationship (see Chapter 8), and a stable overbite.

10.7.2 Overbite is to be corrected

If the overbite is to be corrected and the result remain stable, then the interincisal angle must be changed. Typically, in a class II division 2 incisor relationship the interincisal angle is so high that there is an insufficient occlusal stop to prevent the incisor teeth from erupting past one another. Ideally the interincisal angle should be corrected to an angle of approximately 135° in order to provide this occlusal limitation. Altering the inclination of the upper and lower incisor teeth, without changing the overall anteroposterior position of their crowns, which might adversely affect long term stability, requires the use of upper and lower fixed appliances. Treatment planning should once again begin in the lower arch, with an assessment of the space requirements for alignment of the lower incisors and canines. As with class I and class II division 1 incisor relationships the lower arch may be treated with a fixed appliance with or without extractions, depending upon the degree of crowding present. Occasionally, treatment can be started with non-extraction and the case reassessed following overbite reduction and initial alignment of the teeth. This is known as therapeutic diagnosis and is of use in class II division 2 incisor relationships which are borderline cases for extraction or non-extraction. In some instances, overbite reduction is easily achieved by starting treatment without any extractions, but it is important the patient is informed that extractions may be necessary part way through treatment, following clinical and cephalometric reassessment. Once the lower arch has been planned, treatment of the upper arch is aimed at achieving a class I canine relationship so that a class I incisor relationship can be created and the interincisal angle corrected. The molar relationship will be class I if both the upper and lower arches are treated by a non-extraction technique, or if both are treated by the loss of a premolar unit in each quadrant. The molar relationship will be class II if the lower arch is treated non-extraction and the upper arch is treated by the loss of a premolar unit in each quadrant. Whether headgear is necessary to reinforce upper arch anchorage or distalize the upper buccal segment teeth will depend on the initial molar relationship, as discussed with class I malocclusions. Careful management of the headgear in combination with a fixed appliance can lead to extrusion of the posterior maxillary teeth, assisting in the correction of the overbite.

10.7.3 Presence of severe class II skeletal base

Occasionally, class II division 2 malocclusions present on moderate to severe class II skeletal bases. If the patient is prepubescent, it is possible to procline the upper incisors, creating a class II division 1 incisor relationship, which can then be treated as such with a myofunctional appliance to help correct the anteroposterior skeletal discrepancy. Upper incisor proclination in these patients can sometimes be very difficult, requiring a combination of fixed and removable appliances either before, or as part of the myofunctional appliance therapy. As with class II division 1 malocclusions treated with a myofunctional appliance, such cases may be reassessed at the end of this phase of treatment, to determine whether a second, fixed appliance phase of treatment is necessary, with or without extractions or headgear. Patients with the same moderate to severe skeletal patterns, but who have passed their pubertal growth spurt, may only be treatable by a combination orthodontics and orthognathic surgery. Fixed appliance therapy, with or without extractions, is necessary to decompensate the arches prior to the orthognathic surgery for the underlying anteroposterior skeletal discrepancy.

10.8 CLASS III MALOCCLUSIONS

When planning treatment in Class III malocclusions the major considerations are:

(1) the anteroposterior skeletal pattern

(2) the age of the patient

(3) the potential for further facial growth.

If the skeletal pattern is class I or mild class II, planning treatment in the presence of a class III incisor relationship is usually straightforward. Planning is comparable to that of a class I malocclusion discussed earlier, except that it should begin with the upper arch. This is because it is this arch which is usually the most crowded and the creation of a class I incisor relationship entails proclining the upper incisors into a positive overbite and overjet. Treatment of the lower arch is then planned so that the lower teeth occlude normally with the corresponding upper arch teeth. Once a space analysis has been performed in the upper arch and extractions planned for the relief of crowding, lower arch extractions, where necessary, are then planned. A commonly applied rule is that extractions in the lower arch should match those in the upper arch, or are one tooth further mesially in the arch (i.e. if upper second premolars are extracted then either lower second or lower first premolars are extracted, but if upper first premolars are extracted then only lower first premolars can be extracted). However, this is a general rule and requires assessing each case on its own merits.

Treatment planning may also be relatively straightforward in the presence of a mild class III skeletal base. However, care must be taken when planning treatment for such cases, due to the possible unfavourable effects of continued facial growth. In a case with a class I or class II skeletal base, average increments of facial growth would be expected to maintain or even improve anteroposterior skeletal relations over time. With class III skeletal bases the opposite may be true, so they become instead more severe with continued growth. Care therefore needs to be exercised in treatment planning where a great deal of facial growth is yet to occur and there is a class III skeletal relationship. For example, a child may present at the age of 11 years with a class III incisor relationship and a reverse overjet, which might be readily treatable to class I by proclination of the upper incisors and retroclination of the lower incisors. However, with continued and unfavourable mandibular growth the class III skeletal base may become more severe, leading to relapse of the corrected incisor relationship and the reappearance of a reverse overjet. If the original orthodontic treatment involved loss of four premolar units, one in each quadrant for the relief of upper arch crowding and to permit lower incisor retroclination, the lower arch extraction spaces may reopen totally on relapse of the reverse overjet. The absence of a positive overbite and overjet may lead to the lower incisors moving labially under the influence of the soft tissues. This is made worse by the fact that in many class III malocclusions there is often little initial crowding in the lower arch and extractions would only have been performed to allow the lower incisors to be retroclined for overjet correction. The upper arch is often crowded, which explains why the extraction spaces do not reopen in this arch on relapse of the overjet. Where such relapse occurs, orthodontic treatment alone will not produce a stable result and an orthognathic approach may be required, particularly if the patient is now concerned by the class III skeletal pattern. Orthodontic decompensation prior to surgery will inevitably mean proclining the lower incisors even further to their correct position over the mandibular base ($\overline{1}$MnP 90° ± 5°) with total reopening of the original premolar extraction sites. In some cases, as a consequence of the mechanics used, the space is greater than the original tooth which had been extracted. Following surgery, these extraction sites would then need to be restored using an acid-etched retained bridge or an implant. Caution therefore needs to be exercised when planning treatment on class III skeletal bases where further substantial facial growth is expected. If there is any doubt as to the effect of continued facial growth, treatment should be deferred and the patient reviewed at later date. Otherwise, treatment performed at this time should be restricted to the upper arch only, with or without extractions. Extractions should not be considered in the lower arch. In this way, the effects of any early treatment will not prejudice later treatment planning if the patient then requires orthognathic surgery due to continued and unfavourable facial growth.

Where caution has been exercised in treatment planning, such that the likely final anteroposterior skeletal pattern is known, a major determinant in planning treatment in class III cases is whether the patient is concerned by their skeletal pattern. If they are unhappy and the skeletal pattern is a moderate to severe class III relationship, then an orthognathic approach may be the ideal treatment option. This would be preceded by presurgical orthodontic treatment with fixed appliances to decompensate the dental arches over their respective skeletal bases. Surgery would then be performed on one or both jaws to correct the underlying skeletal discrepancy.

If the patient is happy with their facial appearance and the skeletal pattern is a mild class III, then orthodontic treatment to correct the class III incisor relationship can be planned along the lines of a class I malocclusion. Lower arch extractions, not only for the relief of crowding, but also to permit retroclination of the lower incisors can then be planned, safe in the knowledge that substantial relapse of the final treatment result is not going to occur, since most facial growth has ceased. If on the other hand the skeletal pattern is moderate to severe class III and yet the patient is unhappy with their extra-oral appearance, then there may be no alternative to a combined orthodontic and orthognathic approach to treatment. Correction of the incisor relationship without orthognathic surgery will not be possible. This is because correction would involve excessive proclination and retroclination of the upper and lower incisors respectively. Not only would this be aesthetically unacceptable, but it would lead to unfavourable occlusal loading of these teeth in function. In addition, there may also be a vertical skeletal discrepancy with an associated anterior open bite, meaning that any such anteroposterior tooth movements would be unstable. In these patients, treatment is therefore limited to relief of crowding, alignment of the teeth, and the closure of any residual extraction spaces, usually with fixed appliances. Due to a lack of anteroposterior or vertical overlap of the incisors post-treatment, tooth alignment is unlikely to remain stable and the patient will need to wear retainers on an indefinite and possibly part time basis.

10.9 CONCLUSIONS AND CASE STUDIES

When planning orthodontic treatment for any of the malocclusions, it is worthwhile devising a number plans of varying complexity, ranging from acceptance through to the ideal and usually most complex. This is because numerous factors must be taken into consideration when matching a treatment plan to the needs of a particular patient and their malocclusion. As has been discussed in other chapters, these will include specific dental factors, for example the prognosis of teeth, any ectopic positioning, or developmental absence. Patient factors, namely medical and dental history, as well as social factors, such as ease of travelling for regular appointments and the availability of local orthodontic services, are also important when planning treatment. When deciding on the most appropriate treatment for a patient, the various available options should be discussed with the patient and/or their parents. Simple treatments will often have limited treatment objectives and the risk/benefit analysis, which will inevitably be considered, should be discussed openly with the patient and parent. They must be made aware of the limited objectives in any simplified treatment plan before it is embarked upon. These might include, for example, limited aesthetic improvement or the need for indefinite retention. In this way, they can make an informed choice as to their preferred treatment option, guided by the advice of the clinician. The patient should then understand the level of commitment required, both during active treatment and post-treatment retention, if their orthodontic treatment is to be successful.

The following cases are used to illustrate the planning process and how a range of plans may be devised for any particular malocclusion. An orthodontic 'sieve' is to be found in Appendix 2, which can be used in the general treatment planning process for these cases.

Case 1: Dento-alveolar problems

A patient presents aged 15 years with a class I incisor relationship on a class I skeletal base. The malocclusion is complicated by an unerupted maxillary canine (palatally positioned) and retained deciduous canine. There is 3 mm of upper labial segment spacing.

The treatment options for any unerupted teeth include:

(1) leaving them alone;

(2) extracting the deciduous and/or permanent tooth;

(3) autotransplantation;

(4) surgically exposing and orthodontically extruding them.

The options, as applied to the unerupted maxillary canine in this case, are given below.

Leave alone

There is a small but potential risk of resorption of the maxillary incisor roots if the unerupted tooth is left in position. The presence or absence of resorption can only be monitored by routine radiographs, thus committing the patient to long term X-ray exposure.

Extract the deciduous canine

This has been shown to be the treatment of choice for spontaneous improvement of the unerupted tooth position. Longitudinal studies of the loss of an unerupted maxillary canine show a 'normalization' in over 70 per cent of cases in the late mixed/early dentition phase.[11] However, this patient is older than the preferred age both chronologically and in terms of dental development, that is, not only is she 15 years of age, but the apices of the second molars have closed. Spontaneous improvement would therefore be limited.

Extract the permanent canine

The problem with this option is the limited prognosis of the deciduous canine tooth. This will not only be determined by occlusal factors (deciduous teeth being less well mineralized than permanent teeth and therefore more likely to undergo occlusal attrition) but also by the surgery to remove the permanent canine. In this particular case the aesthetics of the deciduous canine are acceptable and there is little in the way of occlusal attrition.

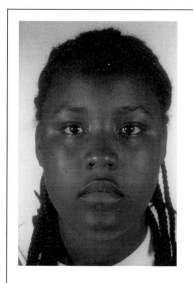
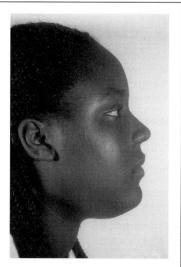
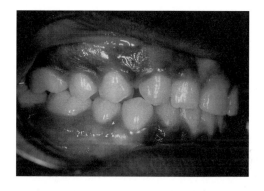
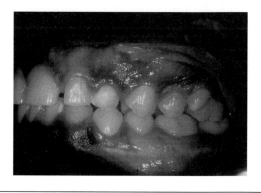

Case 1

Extract both the deciduous and permanent canines

If both teeth are removed and the space closed orthodontically, the lateral incisor/first premolar tooth contact produced is often less than ideal, mainly as a consequence of the smaller mesiodistal dimension of the premolar in comparison with the canine. If the space is retained, then a replacement will be required in the form of an implant or adhesive bridge. A better alternative, in this particular case, than either an implant or bridge would be to leave the deciduous canine in place.

Autotransplantation of the permanent canine

Teeth for transplantation can be considered in two broad categories, depending on the developmental stage of the root:

- open apices
- closed apices

The canine in this case has a closed apex and as such is prone to external root resorption. To prevent this, removal of the pulpal contents is necessary at an early stage and a dressing of calcium hydroxide required to prevent resorption. The long term data on the prognosis of these teeth are limited and a significant proportion are lost after five years. It is not known how such teeth perform in the long term when functioning in canine guidance.

Surgical exposure and orthodontic extrusion

The most reliable treatment for the unerupted canine is exposure followed by the placement of a bonded attachment. In the case of a palatally positioned canine as here, the mucosa is then replaced and the tooth orthodontically extruded over a period of time. Long term results of the replacement of palatal mucosa appear more favourable than in cases where soft tissue is removed. In the case of the buccally positioned unerupted canine, on the other hand, if surgical exposure is required, then an apically repositioned flap is preferred to flap replacement. This ensures that the tooth then erupts through and obtains a gingival margin of attached alveolar mucosa. In the case of the palatally positioned canine in particular, treatment times can easily be underestimated and as a consequence the compliance of the teenage patient tested to the extreme. Following the orthodontic sieve (Appendix 2) in this case:

- Skeletal problem: No
- Dento-alveolar problems requiring orthodontic treatment: options followed depend on patient preference

(Notice the additional buccal cusp on the first molar as a dental abnormality. It does not modify orthodontic treatment but complicates any removable appliance construction.)

Case 1

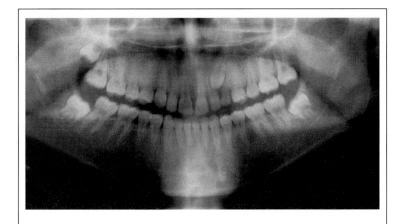

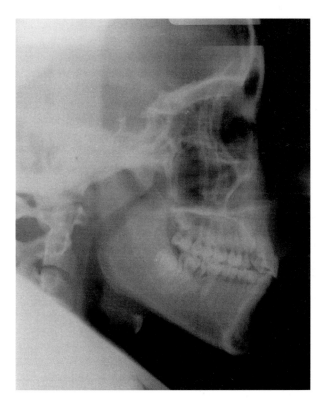

Fig. 10.5 The clinical records for Case 1 used in the diagnosis of an unerupted canine for a patient with dento-alveolar problems.

Case 1

Case 2: A patient with a thumb sucking habit

A boy presents in the mixed dentition stage aged 9 years with a mild class III incisor relationship on a class I skeletal base. There is a marked anterior open bite, a unilateral buccal crossbite, and a lateral displacement of the mandible on closing into centric occlusion. The centre lines are not coincident.

In this case the crossbite is due to a thumb sucking habit which is still continuing, but he is keen to stop.

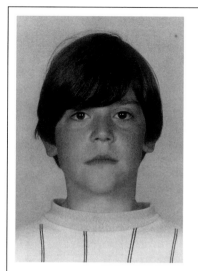
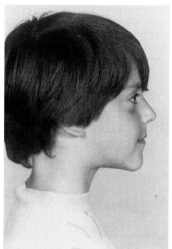

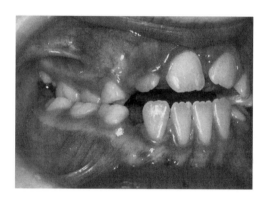

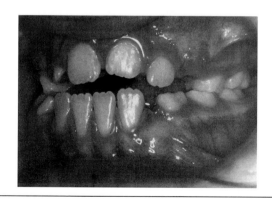

Case 2

The treatment is fairly straightforward, consisting of an upper removable appliance to encourage him to stop thumb-sucking, expanding the upper buccal segments and eliminating the displacement. It should take no longer than six months, but the malocclusion will re-establish itself if the habit does not stop completely.

The orthodontic sieve (Appendix 2) follows the same route as in case 1, above, but this time to 'removable appliance and expansion'.

- Skeletal problem: No
- Dento-alveolar problem requiring ortho only: Yes
- Crowding: Yes
- Removable appl: Expansion

Case 2

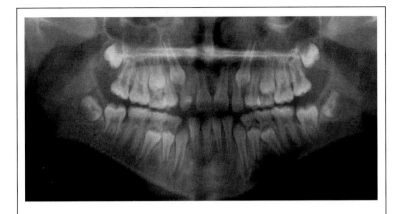

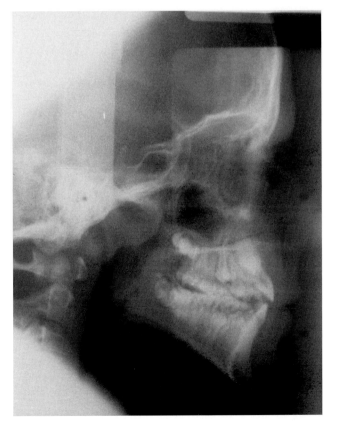

Fig. 10.6   The clinical records of Case 2 with a thumb-sucking habit.

Case 2

Case 3: A class II division 1 camouflage case

This patient presents aged 17 years with a class II division 1 incisor relationship on a class II skeletal base, which is of moderate severity. While the overjet measures 12 mm, it is mainly due to upper incisor proclination. The upper incisor to maxillary plane angle measures 128°. The lower incisors demonstrate dento-alveolar compensation and are proclined.

In this case, the following general assumptions are made.

1. Growth may help to reduce the severity of the skeletal discrepancy, although at 17 years of age the degree of mandibular growth which is still to take place is limited.
2. There is not a functional disorder induced as a consequence of either a class III or a class II molar relationship.

Major points to clarify prior to planning are:

1. At what inclination are the upper incisors?
2. How much palatal bone exists into which the upper incisors can be retracted?
   (a) If the maxillary incisors are at their normal inclination then treatment will be more complex, necessitating fixed appliance therapy at least.
   (b) If the upper incisors are proclined then it may be feasible to correct the increased overjet simply by tipping the upper incisors palatally using an upper removable appliance.

Such a case requires a lateral skull radiograph to be obtained in order to establish the type of treatment required. Again, treatment planning begins with the lower arch teeth (with the exceptions outlined earlier). Once the position of the lower incisors has been planned then the necessary movement of the upper labial segment teeth to create a class I incisor relationship can be determined. Initial assessment of this patient would indicate that the upper incisors have to be retracted in order to create a class I incisor relationship and to completely eliminate the overjet. The upper incisors are already proclined and it is known that upper incisor retraction using a removable appliance will cause these teeth to tip at a point approximately one third from the apex of the root, known as the centroid. By mentally visualizing the rotation about this point using the lateral skull radiograph, the type of appliance required for treatment can be anticipated. If, following the tipping of the upper labial segment the incisors appear to be retroclined, a class II division 2 incisor relationship will be created. This could lead to a deepening of the overbite which might then become traumatic, making the patient worse off at the end of treatment. In many ways it is best to

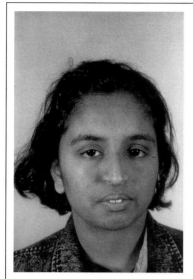
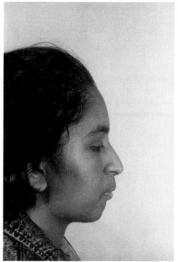
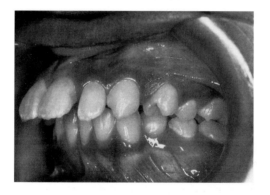
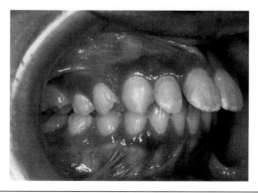

Case 3

establish the treatment as if there were no crowding and to determine the movements required to obtain an ideal incisor relationship. Then, if crowding exists, the extraction pattern can be modified to take this into account.

The sieve identifies a skeletal problem and in this case it was decided to camouflage and retain.

- Skeletal problem: Yes
- Is the patient still growing?: No
- Camoflage and retain

The only other treatment option would be orthodontic decompensation followed by orthognathic surgery.

Case 3

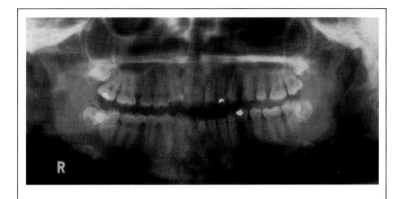

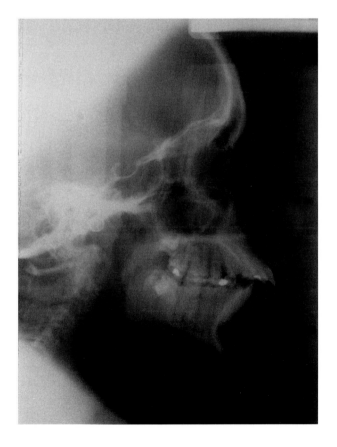

Fig. 10.7 Case 3 presenting a class II division 1 incisor relationship.

Case 3

Case 4: Class II division 2 incisor relationship

This boy aged 15 years presents with a class II division 2 incisor relationship on a mild class II skeletal base. There is a reduced anterior lower face height and the overbite is increased.

Fortunately it is rare for such cases to have a severe skeletal discrepancy and functional appliances in the growing individual or orthognathic surgery are seldom required. Also, by definition, the upper incisors are retroclined and so a removable appliance is not indicated for further retraction of the upper incisors. Removable appliance therapy may be limited to small amounts of distal movement of the upper buccal segments, followed by alignment of the proclined upper lateral incisors. More commonly, fixed appliances are used to reduce the overbite, correct the inter-incisor angle, and to align the teeth. In order to achieve this the upper incisor apices will have to be moved palatally.

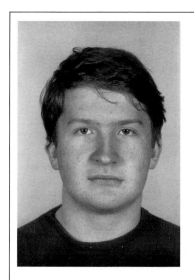
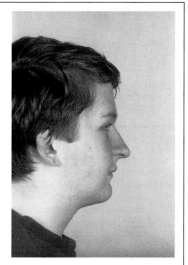
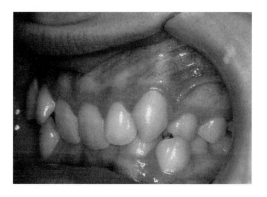
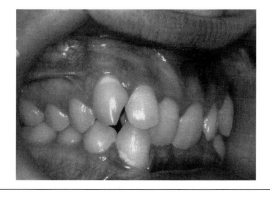

Case 4

This type of malocclusion is often misdiagnosed as being crowded and as a consequence teeth are often extracted at the beginning of the treatment. If there is any doubt as to whether extractions are required, then they can be deferred until mid-way through the fixed appliance therapy. With this technique, known as 'therapeutic diagnosis,' it is important to inform the patient at the start of the fixed appliance therapy that extractions may be necessary later. The final decision on the extractions is usually made after alignment of the teeth and reduction of the overbite (which is easier if no extractions have been performed), and following cephalometric analysis of a mid-treatment lateral skull radiograph.

In this particular case the skeletal discrepancy is indeed mild and the dento-alveolar problems apply. Fixed appliance therapy is indicated for rotational control once the oral hygiene is improved. On no account should teeth be extracted until the operator who will apply the appliances is happy that the need for extraction has been identified.

Using the orthodontic sieve.

- Skeletal problem: No
- Crowding: Yes
- Fixed appl.: Extraction or distal movement – decide during treatment (therapeutic diagnosis)

Case 4

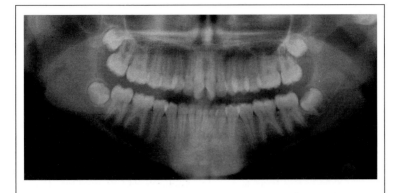

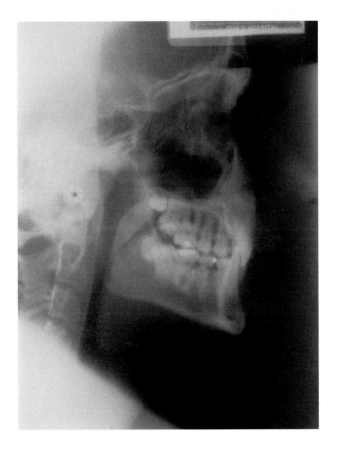

Fig. 10.8 Case 4 showing a class II division 2 incisor relationship.

Case 4

Case 5: Class III case requiring surgery

This patient, aged 14, presents with a class III incisor relationship on a class III skeletal base. There appears to be marked maxillary hypoplasia and retroclined lower incisors.

There is already a history of loss of a premolar unit in the maxilla.

Consider the anteroposterior skeletal pattern, age of the patient, and the potential for further facial growth. If there is any doubt as to stability of orthodontic treatment then it must be totally reversible, so that long term definitive treatment and dental health are not compromised. That is, it is inappropriate to place the teeth into positions which cannot be corrected at a later stage. In particular, the extractions considered may well compromise a surgical treatment later. Therefore, whereas upper arch extractions for the relief of crowding may be permissible, lower arch extractions and complex treatment should be delayed until most facial growth has ceased. In this case further dento-alveolar compensation, in an attempt to create a Class I incisor relationship, would place the teeth into a position of compromised oral health with abnormal inclinations. It would also be unstable. Earlier extractions in the mandibular arch to achieve further retroclination of the lower labial segments would compromise the orthodontic tooth movements required during 'decompensation' prior to orthognathic surgery.

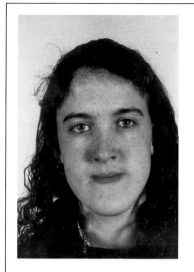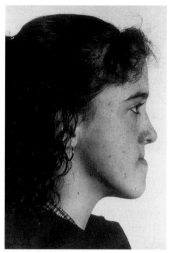

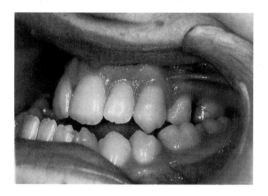

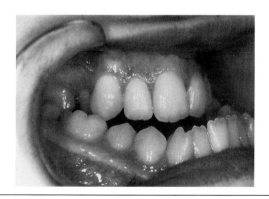

Case 5

In this case facial growth is virtually complete and there should be no doubt that the malocclusion is well beyond the scope of orthodontics alone. Orthognathic surgery will be necessary following orthodontic treatment to decompensate the labial segment teeth and coordinate the dental arches.

Thus from the sieve we have:

- Skeletal problem: Yes
- Is the patient still growing?: Yes
- Skeletal Class III
- Await further growth
- Is there upper arch crowding?: Yes
- Relief of upper arch crowding only +/– appliance
- Accept: No
- Growth complete (approx.)
- Orthodontic decompensation and orthognathic surgery

Case 5

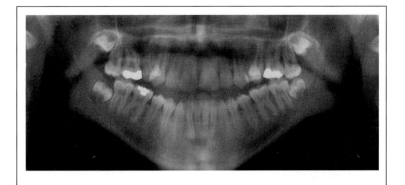

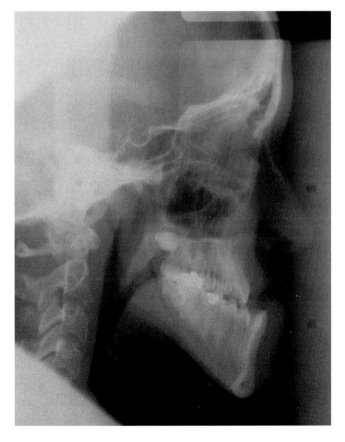

Fig. 10.9   Case 5 presents with a severe class III incisor relationship.

Case 5

Summary

1. Determine the treatment objectives: health, function, aesthetics, and stability.

2. Treatment complexity is based on patient suitability; dento-alveolar factors; skeletal pattern and growth; soft tissues; patient complaints; availability of clinical expertise.

3. Timing of orthodontic treatment. Stages are deciduous dentition, mixed dentition, early permanent dentition, adult dentition.

4. In the early permanent dentition, when most treatment is undertaken, consider each malocclusion.

    (a) Class I: plan lower arch first. Following relief of crowding to align the incisors and create a class I canine relationship, determine the molar relationship, either class I or class II, and how it is to be achieved. It may or may not include extractions, and removable or fixed appliances. Headgear may be required to create space, reinforce the anchorage, or both.

    (b) Class II division 1: check for digit sucking habit. Check skeletal pattern. If it is class I or mild class II skeletal pattern then treat as a class I malocclusion. If it is a moderate to severe skeletal class II then consider a myofunctional appliance during the pubertal growth spurt. If successful, the resulting malocclusion can then be treated, as necessary, like a class I malocclusion, following the myofunctional phase. If the patient is not growing an orthognathic approach may be required or treatment limited to relief of crowding and alignment without overjet correction.

    (c) Class II division 2: whether the overbite is to be accepted or corrected will determine treatment objectives and complexity.

    (d) Class III: consider the anteroposterior skeletal pattern, age of the patient, and the potential for further facial growth. If there is any doubt as to long term stability of orthodontic treatment then it must be totally reversible, so that long term definitive treatment and dental health are not compromised. Whereas upper arch extractions for the relief of crowding may be permissible in such circumstances, lower arch extractions and complex treatment should be delayed until most facial growth has ceased.

REFERENCES

1. Samuels, R. H. A. and Jones, M. L. (1994). Orthodontic facebow injuries and safety equipment. *European Journal of Orthodontics*, **16**, 385–94.
2. Andrews, L. F. (1990). JCO interview: the straight-wire appliance. *Journal of Clinical Orthodontics*, **24**, 493–508.
3. Tanner, J. M., Whitehouse, R. H., Marubini, E., and Resele L. F. (1976). The adolescent growth spurt of boys and girls of the Harpenden growth study. *Annals of Human Biology*, **3**, 109–26.
4. Bradley, J. C. (1976). Age changes in the vascular supply of the mandible. *British Dental Journal* **134**, 142–4.
5. Kjellgren, B. (1948). Serial extraction as a corrective procedure in dental orthopaedic therapy. *Acta Odontologica Scandinavica*, **8**, 17–43.
6. Richardson, A. (1982). Interceptive orthodontics in general dental practice. *British Dental Journal*, **152**, 85–9, 123–7, and 166–70.
7. Clark, W. J. (1982). The twin block traction technique. *European Journal of Orthodontics*, **4**, 129–38.
8. McReynolds, D. C. and Little, R. M. (1991). Mandibular second premolar extraction – postretention evaluation of stability and relapse. *Angle Orthodontist* **61**, 133–44.
9. Christiansen, R. L. and Burstone, C. J. (1969). Centers of rotation within the periodontal space. *American Journal of Orthodontics* **55**, 353–69.
10. Fränkel, R. (1969). The treatment of class II division 1 malocclusion with functional correctors. *American Journal of Orthodontics*, **55**, 265–75.
11. Ericson, S. and Kurol, J. (1988). Early treatment of palatally erupting maxillary canines by extraction of the primary canines. *European Journal of Orthodontics*, **10**, 283–95.

Appendix 1: Pro forma for intra- and extra-oral examination

Diagnostic sheet

Name   Date of birth
Address

- Present Complaint
- Habits   Yes/ No   Thumb/ Finger
- Skeletal Pattern   Antero-posterior   I / II / III   Mild/ Moderate/ Severe
                                 Vertical   FMPA   Average/ Increased/ Decreased
                                                                          MMA   Average/ Increased/ Decreased
                                 Transverse (asymmetry)   Yes/ No

- Soft Tissues   Lips   Competent/ Incompetent
                                 Lip line   High/ Normal/ Low

- Teeth Present   ⊹   • Caries   ⊹

- Tooth quality   Good/ Fair/ Poor   • Hypoplasia   ⊹
- Oral Hygiene   Good/ Fair/ Poor

- Lower labial   Inclination   Average/ Proclined/ Retroclined
  segment   Aligned/ Crowded/ Spaced   Mild/ Moderate/ Severe

- Upper labial   Inclination   Average/ Proclined/ Retroclined
  segment   Aligned/ Crowded/ Spaced   Mild/ Moderate/ Severe
                                 Diastema …..mm

- Overjet   …..mm
- Overbite   Average/ Increased/ Decreased   Complete/ Incomplete/ Traumatic
                                 Anterior open bite …….mm
- Centre lines   Upper - Right/ Central/ Left …..mm
                                 Lower - Right/ Central/ Left …..mm

- Lower buccal segments   Aligned/ Crowded/ Spaced   Mild/ Moderate/ Severe
- Upper buccal segments   Aligned/ Crowded/ Spaced   Mild/ Moderate/ Severe

- Molar relationship   Right   I / II / III $\frac{1}{4}$ / $\frac{1}{2}$ / $\frac{3}{4}$ unit
                                     Left   I / II / III $\frac{1}{4}$ / $\frac{1}{2}$ / $\frac{3}{4}$ unit

- Crossbites   Unilateral - Right/ Left   Displacement - Yes/ No
                                 Bilateral   Displacement - Yes/ No
- Scissors bite   Unilateral/ Bilateral   ⊹

- Radiographs   Upper standard maxillary occlusal
                                 DPT
                                 Lateral skull

- Other investigations

Summary of findings

Appendix 2: Orthodontic 'Sieve'

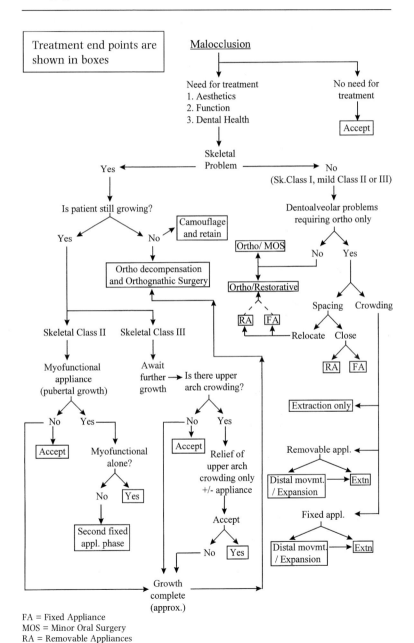

Treatment end points are shown in boxes

Malocclusion

Need for treatment
1. Aesthetics
2. Function
3. Dental Health

No need for treatment

Accept

Skeletal Problem — No (Sk.Class I, mild Class II or III)

Yes

Is patient still growing?

Yes   No

Camouflage and retain

Dentoalveolar problems requiring ortho only

Ortho/ MOS

Ortho decompensation and Orthognathic Surgery

Ortho/Restorative

No   Yes

RA   FA

Spacing   Crowding

Relocate   Close

Skeletal Class II   Skeletal Class III

RA   FA

Myofunctional appliance (pubertal growth)

Await further growth → Is there upper arch crowding?

No   Yes

Extraction only

No   Yes

Accept

Accept   Myofunctional alone?

Relief of upper arch crowding only +/- appliance

Removable appl.

No   Yes

Distal movmt. / Expansion → Extn

Second fixed appl. phase

Accept

Fixed appl.

No   Yes

Distal movmt. / Expansion → Extn

Growth complete (approx.)

FA = Fixed Appliance
MOS = Minor Oral Surgery
RA = Removable Appliances

Appendix 3: Questions

1. Describe the changes which occur in the dentition between 6 and 12 years. What are the possible causes of late lower incisor crowding?

2. Discuss the role of skeletal pattern in the aetiology of malocclusion. Describe briefly how skeletal pattern is assessed.

3. Discuss the importance of the patient/parent interview. What are the different types of consent?

4. How do the soft tissues influence tooth position? What is their significance in orthodontic treatment planning?

5. Discuss the aetiology and possible management of a wide median diastema.

6. Displacements and deviations of the mandible on closing into centric occlusion can be seen in a number of malocclusions. Describe how they are assessed and their significance in orthodontic treatment planning.

7. What are the indications for orthodontic treatment?

8. Describe the various types of orthodontic records and their purpose.

9. What is meant by evidence based practise? Describe its importance in planning lower incisor position.

10. Discuss the significance of timing of orthodontic treatment in class III incisor relationships.

Glossary

Abrasion: The loss of tooth substance as a consequence of wear induced by dissimilar materials such as pumice.

Adaptive swallowing behaviour: This is the swallowing behaviour which is identified when a normal lip to lip anterior oral seal cannot be achieved. Examples include a tongue to lower lip and lower lip to palate anterior oral seal.

Alveolar process: The parts of the maxilla and mandible, the development and existence of which depend on the presence of the teeth. It contains the sockets of erupted teeth and the crypts of developing teeth.

Anchorage: The sites which provide resistance to the reaction generated by the forces applied to move certain teeth. These sites can include other teeth (intra-oral) or they may be extra-oral. It is a concept which can be considered in three directions – anteroposterior, lateral, and vertical.

Angle's classification: A classification of malocclusion based on arch (first molar) relationship in the sagittal plane.

Angulation: The mesiodistal tip of a tooth within the dental arch.

Anterior open bite: The lower incisors are not overlapped in the vertical plane by the upper incisors and do not occlude with them.

Anterior oral seal: A seal normally produced by contact between the lips.

Attrition: The loss of tooth substance as a consequence of tooth wear.

Bimaxillary: Pertaining to both upper and lower dento-alveolar processes.

Buccal segments: The canine, premolar, and molar teeth.

Centric occlusion: A position of maximum intercuspation.

Centric relation: The relationships between the mandible and maxilla when the condyles are in retruded unstrained positions in the glenoid fossae.

Centroid: An imaginary point in the root of a tooth, approximately one third from its apex, about which a tooth will tip when a point force is applied to the crown.

Competent lips: A lip seal is maintained with minimal muscular effort when the mandible is in the rest position.

Complete overbite: An overbite in which the lower incisors make contact with either the upper incisors or the palatal mucosa.

Crossbite: This can either be **anterior** in which case one or more upper incisors are in lingual occlusion with the lower incisors, or **posterior** in which case there is a transverse discrepancy of the buccal segment teeth with one or more upper teeth occluding more palatally than normal.

Dental bases: The maxilla and mandible excluding the alveolar processes.

Dental base relationship: The relationship between the dental bases, with the mandible in the rest position, in any of the three planes of space.

Dento-alveolar adaptation: The changes in angulation/inclination of teeth in their alveolus as a consequence of normal growth and development. This is a **dynamic** process and requires serial records (clinical or radiographic) to identify this change. A typical example would include retroclination of the lower labial segment in a mild class III skeletal relationship as the mandible continues to grow forwards.

Dento-alveolar compensation: This is a **static** phenomenon seen usually on one lateral skull radiograph where the upper and lower labial segment teeth are inclined to 'camouflage' the underlying skeletal base. Typically the lower incisors may be proclined and the upper incisors of normal inclination in a patient with a class II skeletal base. This will result in the overjet not being a reflection of the underlying skeletal base discrepancy.

Deviation of the mandible: A sagittal movement of the mandible during closure from a habit posture to a position of centric occlusion.

Diastema: A space between certain teeth, often maxillary central incisors.

Dilaceration: The deformed development of a tooth often as a result of the disturbance by trauma of the uncalcified and calcified portions of the developing tooth.

Disclusion: The dynamic separation of opposing teeth during mandibular movements.

Displacement of the mandible: A sagittal or lateral movement of the mandible from the rest position to the position of maximum intercuspation as a result of a premature occlusal contact.

Displacement (tooth): The malposition of the crown and the root of an individual tooth to an equal degree and in the same direction. Often prefixed by mesio, disto, bucco, labio, linguo, supra, or infra to describe the direction.

Erosion: The loss of tooth substance as a consequence of chemical dissolution as found from dietary excesses.

Freeway space: The space between the occlusal surfaces of the teeth when the mandible is in the rest position or a position of habitual posture.

Ideal occlusion: A theoretical occlusion based on the morphology of the teeth.

Imbrication: The overlapping of incisor teeth in the same arch.

Inclination: The labiopalatal tip of a tooth within the dental arch (also labiolingual/buccopalatal/buccolingual).

Incisors, lingual surface of upper: Divided into three parts as follows: (1) the acutely inclined surface from the incisal tip, with an average angle of 4° to the long axis; (2) the cingulum plateau on average 30° to the long axis; (3) the cervical part extending to the gingival margin at an angle of 6° to the long axis.

Incisor classification: A classification based on the incisor relationship in the sagittal plane.

Incompetent lips: With the mandible in the rest position the lips are apart and muscular effort is required to obtain a lip seal.

Incomplete overbite: An overbite in which the lower incisors contact neither the upper incisors nor the palatal mucosa.

Intermaxillary space: The space between the upper and lower dental bases when the mandible is in the rest position.

Interocclusal clearance: This is the space between the upper and lower dentitions.

Labial segments: The incisor teeth.

Leeway space: The excess space provided when the deciduous canine and molars are replaced by the permanent canine and premolars. The leeway space is slightly greater in the lower arch.

Malocclusion: An occlusion in which there is a malrelationship between the arches in any of the three planes of space or in which there are anomalies in tooth position beyond the limits of acceptable 'norm'.

Non-working side: This is the side away from which the mandible moves during normal masticatory function.

Normal occlusion: An occlusion which satisfies the requirements of function and aesthetics but in which there are minor irregularities of individual teeth.

Overjet: The relationship between the upper and lower incisors in the horizontal plane.

Overbite: The overlap of the lower incisors by the upper incisors in the vertical plane.

Posterior oral seal: A seal between the soft palate and dorsum of the tongue.

Postured position: A position of the mandible habitually maintained either to facilitate the production of an anterior oral seal or for aesthetic reasons.

Premature contact: An occlusal contact which occurs during the centric path of closure of the mandible before maximum intercuspation. This may result in either a displacement of the mandible, movement of the tooth, or both.

Primate spacing: A naturally occurring space in the deciduous dentition, mesial to the upper canine and distal to the lower canine.

Proclined: The upper or lower incisors are inclined labially to a greater degree than normal.

Prognathism: The projection of the jaws from beneath the cranial base.

Rest position of the mandible: The position of the mandible in which the muscles acting on it show minimal activity. Essentially it is determined by the resting lengths of the muscles of mastication.

Retroclined: The upper or lower incisor are inclined palatally/lingually to a greater extent than normal. Words such as 'upright' or 'vertical' are confusing and should be avoided.

Scissors bite: One or more upper buccal segment teeth occlude entirely buccal to the lower arch teeth.

Skeletal pattern: The relationship between the dental bases in the sagittal plane.

Supernumerary teeth: Teeth in excess of the usual number, and usually of abnormal form.

Supplemental teeth: Supernumerary teeth, resembling teeth of the normal series.

Working side: During normal masticatory function it is the side to which the mandible shifts.

Index